Polyvagal Theory

A Beginner's Guide to Understand How Trauma Affects the Body

Gabriel Davidson

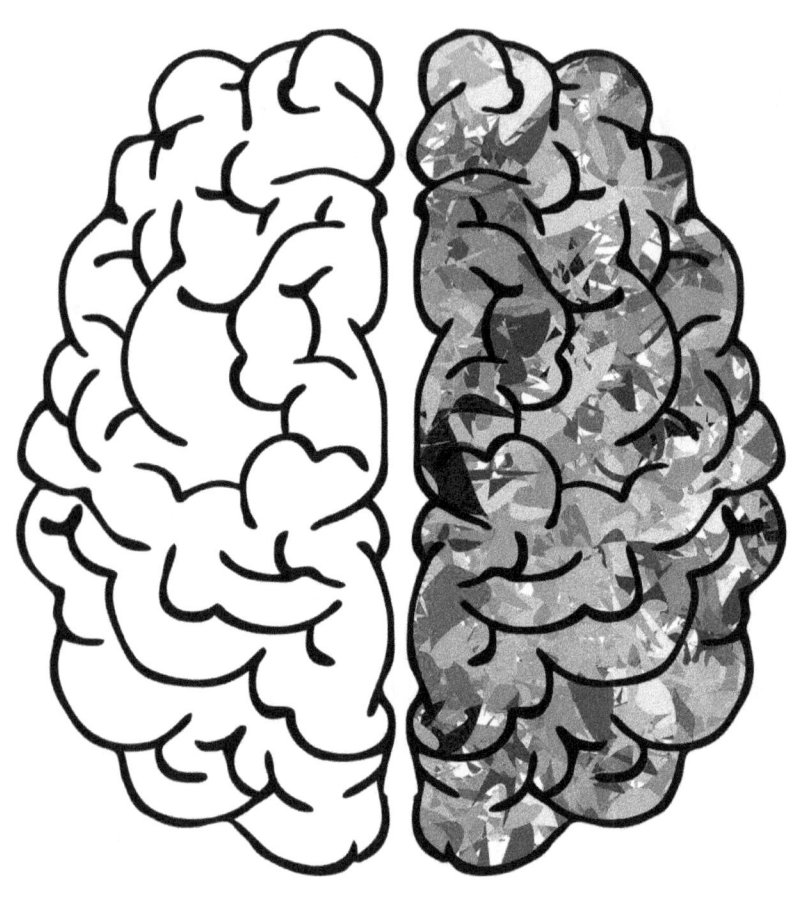

©Copyright 2021 - *Gabriel Davidson* - All rights reserved

The content contained within this book may not be reproduced, duplicated, or transmitted without direct written permission from the author or the publisher.

Under no circumstances will any blame or legal responsibility be held against the publisher, or author, for any damages, reparation, or monetary loss due to the information contained within this book, either directly or indirectly.

Legal Notice

This book is copyright protected. This book is only for personal use. You cannot amend, distribute, sell, use, quote or paraphrase any part, or the content within this book, without the consent of the author-publisher.

Disclaimer Notice

Please note the information contained within this document is for educational and entertainment purposes only. All effort has been executed to present accurate, up to date, and reliable, complete information. No warranties of any kind are declared or implied. Readers acknowledge that the author is not engaging in the rendering of legal, financial, medical, or professional advice.

Table of Contents

Introduction 5

Chapter 1: What is Polyvagal Theory 9

    Application of polyvagal Theory 21

Chapter 2: Importance of Polyvagal Theory 27

Chapter 3: The polyvagal Activities and Mind & Body Activities 33

Chapter 4: The Impact of Nervous System on Our Bodies 46

    Understanding the Autonomic Nervous System? 48

Chapter 5: Dealing with Autism and Mental Stress 61

    Mental Stress and Polyvagal Theory 77

Chapter 6: Trauma Experiences and Polyvagal Theory 82

    Effect of Trauma On Nervous System And Its Response 94

Conclusion 98

Introduction

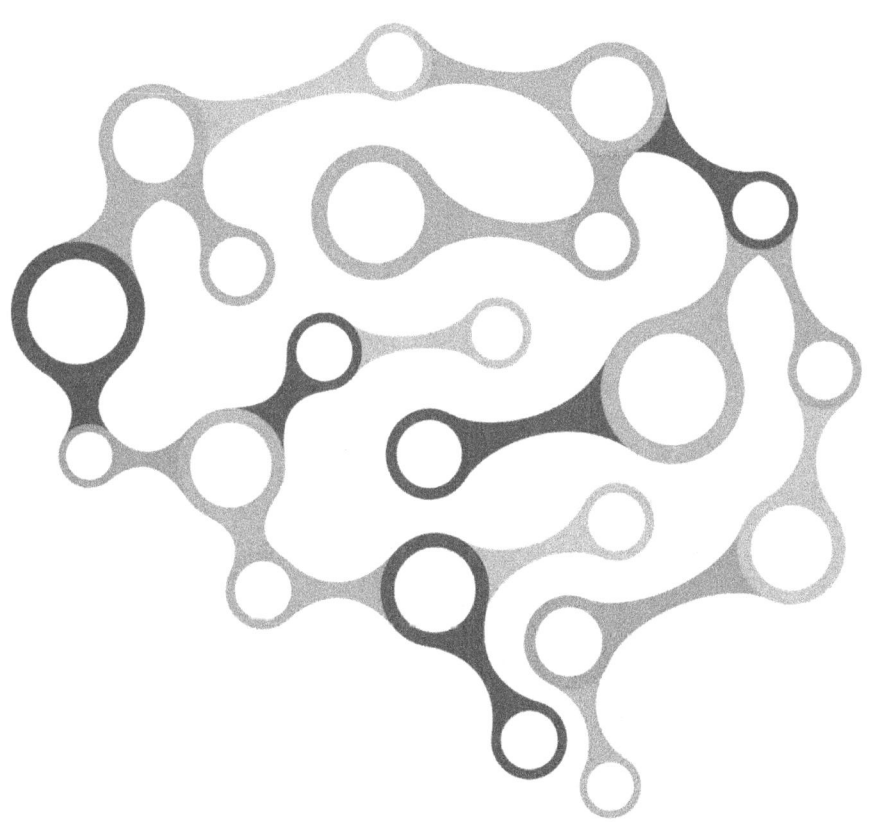

We all hope for a smooth life throughout. No one anticipates experiencing some breakdowns and low moments in life. We face each day filled with positive vibes, hoping for the best. However, that is always not the case. At times, we face difficult situations whereby people, events, relationships, abuse, and traumatic experiences live leave us in an emotional breakdown situation. In the end, we feel low and have a mental breakdown. Even if the time passed by and we recall, it feels like passing through that repeatedly, which reawaken memories, and switching states feels like hell. Some people are so toxic and judgmental that they always keep judging, taunting, making comments, misguiding, calling names, and hurting others. They stay busy letting others down; if they started feeling how others feel about such acts, they would never do that again.

Some situations can be tough to imagine because they dump us into an emotional position that can't go away. On hurting expectations, our minds could stay in the situation for months and even years. Our immaturity is also a significant reason for uncertain circumstances. We start giving our full potential, and we get involved with all our hearts and soul to fake and toxic people. These friendships and relations break our trust and entirely shatter us. In the end, such happenings push us into trauma, and we feel like the entire world has turned against us.

We end up as broken human beings in terms of physical, emotional, and mental states. It is okay to feel the pressure and face some psychological symptoms and engage ourselves in deep thoughts. You can sometimes experience sleepless nights, procrastination, crying, and other related problems bothering your thoughts. The results are unhappy souls, depressed people, anxiety, and loneliness feelings.

All these happenings within our bodies affect our brains primarily. And since the brain is a crucial organ in our body, most functionalities stop affecting our overall health. That is how stress issues come in, leading to high blood pressure, obesity, diabetes, and other related diseases. Repetitive stress and traumas affect our moods, expertise, food intake and bring on anxiety disorders. The impact of trauma on the mind is commonly the foremost distressing. Traumatic events leave us feeling insecure. They disrupt our beliefs and assumptions concerning the world. The sense of ability to manage our life could also be shattered. Elements of the brain will become supersensitized, inflicting us to get on high alert and understand threats worldwide, leaving us anxious and stressed.

In the end, our bodies become weak, unable to respond to daily activities. When people and situations break us, nature helps our bodies to heal us. It is the self-sufficiency, our nervous system, and its responses that react, work against it, fight for us, settles everything, and make us feel better, even more, better than we were used to be. The body's response plays a critical role in dealing with stress and danger in our environment.

Our bodies then prepare to fight and deal with such conditions.

That is why theories such as polyvagal theory explain the happenings to the autonomic nervous system. The purpose of the nervous system in our bodies is to build connections among the body organs. That is why polyvagal theory and how the body responds to traumatic experiences are related aspects. As you read on, you will unleash more details about the theory.

Chapter 1:
What is Polyvagal Theory

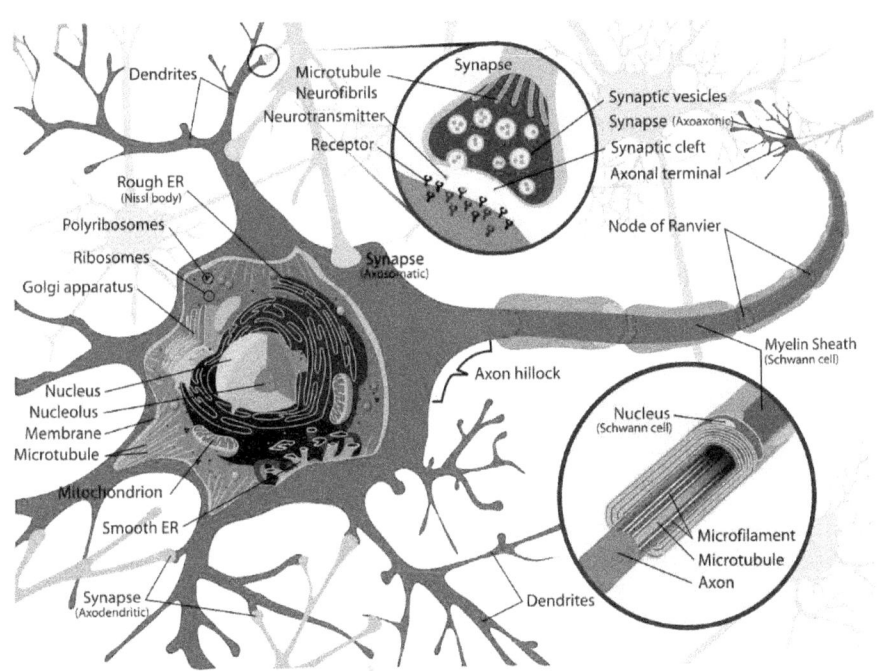

The medullary source, which is the brain stem medulla, boasts diverse capacities typical of the vagus nerve. For a proper understanding of most, if not all, various degrees, the Polyvagal theory is essential. The idea aims at pointing out two major working branches of the vagus nerve. The stems are split further into two classes: the dorsal motor nuclei or simply DMNX and the nucleus ambiguous abbreviated as NA. Therefore, the theory plays a valuable role in understanding how the vagus nerve's parasympathetic coordination of a range of organs relates to or connects to the visceral activity.

Before the Polyvagal theory came into existence at the initial stages, there was a different perception of the nervous system. The system was initially believed to be a two-part antagonistic system. However, the Polyvagal theory stretches to the different extent of exploring the social engagement system, a third response of the nervous system.

Stephen Porges' Theory

Among the renowned psychiatry professors, you wouldn't miss out on Stephen Porges, a known professor who's currently from North Carolina University. Professor Stephen Porges boasts some of the critical achievements which earned him better tittles that define him as a great university scientist. Among his most outstanding establishments at Indiana University is consortium research on traumatic stress. Some of his most incredible developments don't just confine to a few kinds of research. Still, it is also essential to understand that through him, we can define the effects of visceral occurrences on the nervous system and the accompanying human behavior in what is called the Polyvagal theory. It is one of the most fantastic ideas incorporating a unique and fresh perspective into the link between action and autonomic function. It is a unique perspective that aims to define the autonomic system as its central body system. The theory explores an in-depth focus on neural circuits that convert into autonomic reactivity, which lies in the sub-area of the mammalian autonomic nervous system's phylogeny. One of the most fantastic subjects or points of focus of this theory is an extensive understanding of the autonomic nervous system, including efferent and afferent pathways and the objective organ. In this case, the former path serves the vital role of relaying messages from the brain to the body while the latter vice versa. The theory, too, ensures comprehension of the two-way communication and mutual effects between the heart (an organ) and the central nervous system.

It also goes to a different extent of conclusion, justification, and paradigm analysis. All these roles conjunctively establish the theory's central role in the autonomic system in social behavior regulations. Therefore, the Polyvagal theory offers a comprehensive approach to the highlighted areas. Consequently, we can consider it's changing from time to time because of the neuropsychological enhancements that result in the recreation of more recent models, hence expanding the Polyvagal theory.

Another significant consideration under the Polyvagal theory is regulating survival-oriented behaviors through the brain structures' phylogenetic origins. It also incorporates an understanding of the hierarchical responses created into the autonomic nervous system as they link vertebrate animal evolutions. One of this theory's more straightforward objectives is to highlight how the physiological state establishes several psychological experiences and the physiological state's role in establishing the spectrum of behavior. It provides a potential explanation of the communication, social and emotional behaviors, and disorders and ensures concrete highlighting reasons behind responses resulting from stress. For you to draw distinctive features or roles between the physiological and anatomic perspectives of each branch of the vagus nerve, the theory ensures to focus on each unit intensely.

Furthermore, it highlights a proposition for correlation between the two branches through a particular behavior-related strategy. It also tries to expand the three phylogenetic stages in the mammalian autonomic nervous system's evolution process. We can understand three critical subsystems; each follows a phylogenetic order and depicts mobilization, immobilization, and communication correlations.

Therefore, the subsystems include the parasympathetic and

sympathetic branches and ventral vagal pathways, a recent top-up on the units. The parasympathetic branch, also known as the dorsal vagal pathway, responds to immobilization and serves as one of the earliest and most primitive paths.

It has a significant dependence on the vegetative vagus nerve. The sympathetic and ventral vagal pathways take care of mobilization response and carry communication, social and behavioral engagement patterns that confine to unique mammalian species. Each subsystem adopts a unique approach or strategy just efficient to itself.

Therefore, the phylogenetic order of the autonomic nervous system is a summary of the following classifications:

1. The dorsal vagal complex responsible for immobilization
2. The sympathetic nervous system for mobilization
3. Ventral vagal complex responsible for communication, emotion, and motion

The Dorsal Vagal Complex

The subsystem predominantly deals with mammalian hypoxic responses, digestive and taste reactions. For Dorsal Vagal Complex, the efferent nerve fibers' source is the DMNX, dorsal motor nucleus of the vagus nerve. On the other hand, the main afferent vagal counterpart ends at the heart of the solitary tract. The function dorsal vagal complex relates to vestigial roles in humans. Reduced oxygen or hypoxia can trigger the DVC to a greater extent. It is one of the deadliest occurrences in mammals, even though the reptiles can survive under such conditions. The DVC ensures to control the tone of the gut and enhance the digestive processes. However, it should be noted that the same occurs under usual physiological conditions. The DVC is also significant under certain terrible or threatening health conditions. For instance, pathophysiological conditions such as ulcers, to some extent, cool down after a regulatory action through the DVC. The Dorsal Vagal Complex is the last "savior" during certain health anomalies. Therefore, if any other systems fail, the DVC dissociates, goes down, and the following action is a shutdown of the autonomous nervous system.

The Sympathetic Nervous System

Another essential subsystem is the Sympathetic Nervous System. It serves a more significant role in preparing the body to tackle emergencies, increasing breathing rate, inhibiting gastrointestinal activities, and enhancing skin protection through sweat gland stimulation. Experts also believe in its relation to emotion and stress.

The Ventral Vagal Complex

One of the latest and probably the last developments of the phylogenetic order is the Ventral Vagal Complex(VVC). Some of the standard components of these latest developments include the visceromotor and somatomotor features. The efferent fibers of this development start from the nucleus ambiguous. Contrarily, its afferent fibers end at the source of nuclei of the trigeminal and facial nerves. The vagal pathway sourcing from the nucleus ambiguous, running all through to the heart's sinoatrial node, and the bronchi have sheath insulation to ensure the efficiency role. The role of the insulation is to provide increased efficiency in the transmission of nerve signals. Both the somatomotor and the visceromotor components have more significant roles to play. The former ensures proper control and modulation of behaviors essential for a deep dig-up of the social environment. The latter plays a vital role in regulating the bronchi's vagal power (effective organ for providing metabolic resources within a social setting) and the heart.

Stanley Rosenberg's Theory

You probably must have come across this theory too. It is one other grand theory instituted by Stanley Roseburg, a body therapist and author. Stanley hails from America (his birthplace) with the great experience of rolfing since 1983. The author has also taken part in craniofacial therapies for around 34 years ago. Stanley took his 7-year biochemical radiotherapy course at Alain Gehim. He further advanced knowledge in his preferred study area by taking a craniosacral therapy course at the Upledger Institute. His study history is broad and doesn't confine only to therapeutic areas: he also partook in some osteopathy courses at Jean-Pierre Barral. Roseburg also served a few years as a structural integration teacher, visceral massage, biotesegrity, biochemical craniosacral therapy, and much more.

As a top-up of his essential duties, he served typical roles such as yoga instructing, voice training, and acrobatic instructing. He is among the most outstanding scholars who incorporate the polyvagal theory as a potential healer of various health issues such as:

- Migraine headaches
- Anxiety and panic attacks
- Bipolar disorders
- Shoulder, head, and neck aims
- Post-traumatic stress disorders
- Chronic obstructive pulmonary disease and Hiatal hernias, among other typical but crucial health complications.

Chronic obstructive pulmonary disease (COPD) and Hiatal Hernias

The world currently suffers greater threats from many specific diseases. Among these diseases is COPD. Several symptoms are evident, especially when you have contracted COPD. Some of the most common ones include coughing, poor airflow, and shortness of breath. Some of the common causes of this disease include dangerous exposures to environmental toxins, smoking, etc. if one smokes or gets exposed to environmental toxins, there is a greater potential that the body will react to each form of exposure. For instance, in this case, the body reacts by laying down extra bronchiole and lung fibers, which gradually narrows the air pathways. If such occurs, then there is a great potential that the individual facing the same will suffer breathing difficulties. As a remedy, individuals facing similar conditions rely on inhalers and steroids. The two open up and clear the airways but don't guarantee to clear the condition completely: the symptoms may revive after the drug wears off with time. Roseburg, in his thinking, believes that problems linked to COPD emanate from autonomic nervous system dysfunction. Therefore, he goes to a greater extent of incorporating the Polyvagal theory to solve the health problem. Consequently, he considers treatment through various approaches: one being the functional restoration of the vagus nerve.

On the other hand, a hiatal hernia occurs when the stomach gets pulled up against the diaphragm. Such a situation or condition occurs with gradual shortening or tightening of the esophagus. It enlarges the small diaphragm opening bringing about a stomach's pull-up into the chest cavity when such happens. The health condition occurs in the case of vagal dysfunction. Therefore, a correlation between the ventral branch of the vagus nerve and the upper part of the esophagus brings about the possibility of vagal dysfunction. Victims of this condition suffer breathing difficulties or heartburn.

Shoulder, Neck, and Head Pain
Once in a while, you might experience these typical health conditions after perhaps some strenuous activity. However, it isn't

the case, as always. Among the most significant muscles situated in the neck and shoulder are the sternocleidomastoid and trapezius, respectively. The spinal accessory nerve is responsible for innervating the two muscles. If the spinal accessory nerve (CN XI) experiences some complications, stiffness and pain strike both the shoulder and neck regions. Frequent exercises and workouts help reduce or eliminate muscle pains and tension and, as a general role, improves the vagal nerve (CN X) functionality role. Both the spinal accessory nerve and the vagal nerve hold onto a close relationship, with both serving as cranial nerves essential for social engagement.

Migraine Headaches

According to some research statistics, the possible causes of migraines are not yet defined. While most of them are common among people, it is hard to establish possible treatments. As researchers define solutions to headaches as unestablished, people explore a range of options to find some of the potential causes of the health complication to get possible solutions. For instance, some consider migraines as a result of psychological conditions. Some of the psychological states associated with headaches include anxiety, bipolar disorder, among others. Incorporating the Polyvagal theory in such health shortcomings derives a reliable interest. To relieve migraines for some time, Stanley considers tension release in the sternocleidomastoid muscles and the trapezius in the pertinent trigger points. He also believes the improvement of the vagal dysfunction is an improvement for the same.

Bipolar Disorder

An alternation between periods of depressive behaviors and emotional highs generates a given pattern of behavior. The pattern is what we can define as Bipolar disorder. Usually, euphoria and elation periods occur successively with depression and low energy periods. In this case, incorporating polyvagal theory helps us understand how the euphoric state comes about as a stimulation of the spinal sympathetic chain.

Post-Traumatic Stress Disorder

The human nervous system is so pliable that it can easily bounce back after traumatic occurrences. If a Post-Traumatic Disorder occurs, there is a great possibility that the affected individuals may not remain in a state of chronic stress. However, according to various studies, the victim may suffer depression since the healthy

Ideally, humans possess a resilient autonomic nervous system, which often bounces back after a traumatic occurrence. In the case of PTSD, trauma leaves a person not in a state of chronic stress but in a state of dorsal vagal activity, which results in depression. Self-regulation is one of the characteristics of the autonomic system. Therefore, a safe environment depicts that we will enjoy relaxed bodies with great potential for social engagement.

Anxiety and Panic Attacks

Anxiety is a common occurrence in daily life. It comes in different ways, especially during an encounter with challenging decision-making in major life situations—usually, most disorders associated with anxiety always couple up with some worries and fear. If an individual suffers from anxiety disorders at one point or another, there is great potential that the disorder may not vanish away immediately. Some cases of anxiety stick into a person and even get worse from time after time. With consistency in things that generate fear and worries among individuals, we expect that such individuals experience meddles and effects in their day-to-day activities. The outcome is a reduction in productivity, which generally lowers the economy. Psychologically, fear is a process that results in immobilization through the dorsal vagal center. It can also bring about mobilization in the sympathetic chain. In the case of fear attacks, there is an increase in the release of stress hormones, which increases the heartbeat rate and breathing rate. Too, anxiety results in a mixture of worrying thoughts that affect the mind chronically by plaguing it. Short terror and uncertainty moments serve as panic attacks on the victim. Usually, panic attacks occur certainly and end up peak up within shorter periods. The victims can counter such attacks through regular exercises or any other simpler techniques to save the victim from sympathetic nervous system activation or dorsal vagal activation to social communication and engagement.

Application of polyvagal Theory

The polyvagal theory has a great role in undertaking the most crucial situations that demand practical applications. Therefore, the theory has a range of practical applications that cut across various subfields. Practical applications of this theory often result in the most crucial remedies of some critical health anomalies. It is a potential source of enhancing social management because we can highlight, understand and explore social connections. It is reliable for guidance through body-altering to shift between a range of parts of the nervous system. The polyvagal theory is a general guide that will help you understand every action you take in your body, your interactivity with the world around you, and how you can adjust your interaction with the environment or world around you.

This section will touch on the four ways in which the Polyvagal theory is essential to you or any other person. You will often encounter the theory in critical instances such as social connection, stress management, etc.

The Polyvagal Theory and Stress Management

According to the Polyvagal theory, stress management occurs through activation of the vagus nerve. Your decisions on the perception of the environment around you often rely on the vagus nerve. The nerve, too, helps you decide how you would react to any form of stimuli around you. It is your clear guide for everything you undertake in daily life. According to the theory, you have three crucial ways of handling anything in your life. The three ways include calmness and shutting down, being highly alert, and being balanced between the prior states. Usually, looking at stress experiences triggers defense mechanisms such as freeze and shutdown response and fight or flight mechanism. Threats often result in such defensive mechanisms. During stress periods, the vagus nerve is responsible for triggering these defensive mechanisms. During such occurrences, it is essential to understand what prevails through some of the common responses. The responses often result in the onset of effective changes. To understand each of the processes that occur, you first have to take control of the situation.

Therefore, the Polyvagal theory helps us understand the need for entire response control without leaving it at the understanding level. Therefore, it is critical to consider self-nervous activation to easily adjust our minds to a settled state. It is an essential process as you will understand time after time requirements depending on your current model. You will also understand what action to take to achieve the state you need to be in.

The Polyvagal Theory and Social Connection

Through the Polyvagal theory, we can also understand the social connection. The theory addresses the idea that there is a need to be in a given state of mind for anyone to interact happily with people. For instance, interacting with people happily demands some extent of relaxation. To achieve a desired social connection state, you have to take the right neurological activation and the right mental state. Using the right neurological activation calls for a relaxed mental state. It demands getting rid of typical freedom from anxiety, stress. Activation also requires that you get free from alertness to activate the ventral vagal's functioning, requiring you to fall into social engagement. For you to activate the social engagement system, you have to first relax.

Being in this activation means calmness and enables better socialization with people around. The ventral vagal nerve innervating in the middle ear is the possible source of this kind of activation. The activation also possibly comes from facial muscles and the larynx. It is logical because the social engagement system and the process of activation help you socialize with others. Background noise filtrations often go along with the middle ear innervation and activation, helping us achieve focus on interactions. It is also essential to note that the vagus nerve is responsible for activation within the facial muscles and, in the process, enables proper communication through expressions. For the larynx, innervating enables the vagus nerve to alter the voice hence instituting proper interactions, soothing and social speaking. Being in one of those other activations, the fight, flight, or freeze response, possibly marks the beginning of escaping from it through the social engagement system. For instance, individuals in such states can consider engaging in socialization without feeling part of the experience through the fight or flight response. Living happily becomes a reality once we convince and ensure ourselves some safety. It, in turn, helps us stay active in the social engagement system.

Using Top-Down Methods to Influence the Body and Mind

The top-down methods are crucial in helping us emerge from periods of stressed mind states. It is a great way of influencing the body and mind to react in the right way. The methods will enable you to alter your body's feeling by hand in hand with the state of mind. Practically, a calm state of mind generates calmness in the entire body. Calming your mind, therefore, helps you to manage yourself effectively. One of the best approaches to take is to talk yourself down from a situation. For instance, consistent assurance that you don't need to get afraid as there isn't anything to get afraid of in the first place. Doing so also requires that you take yourself through steps to why you believe in your safety, the assurance of your safety, and awareness of the current feelings. To achieve such, you require meditation and mindfulness to find mind calmness that later extends to the body in general. Activating mindful responses occurs through distancing yourself from activities that can otherwise interrupt your mind in one way or the other. It also helps you counter negativity to assure yourself more safety, happiness, and general body control. In this book, we shall cover mindfulness as a way of triggering your vagus nerve.

Using Bottom-Up Methods to Influence the Body and Mind

Apart from the top-bottom approach, the bottom-up methods are also crucial in influencing the mind and body. The method enables you to find precise means or methods of altering the body to change the current mental state. For instance, when you feel stressed and anxious, you may have the mindset that nothing can make you feel anxious. However, there are instances where you may fail to handle the sensation that something is wrong. Such moments come with terrific experiences that you have to establish some of the crucial ways to find solutions. One better approach to counter such situations is faking it until you make it. Understanding and exploring all the possible body languages of the exact feeling you want for yourself is crucial and serves as the onset of picking up naturally. For instance, you can consider every kind of action that would not happen during stress. For instance, considering actions like salivating can be helpful because your mind relies on it and will consider that it cannot get stressed because of a simple action like salivating.

Usually, your mouth contrarily becomes dry during instances of fright or fear, or stress. Therefore, if you use your breathing exercises properly, you will likely achieve many advantageous outcomes in countering stress or any form of fear. First, your body recognizes the action you are trying to take as slowing down and can't get possible stress during deep breathing. From a general aspect, the mind should at least not think of what is happening. Therefore, using your vagus nerve to set yourself free from stress responses requires trying either the top-down or bottom-up approach. Each approach is suitable depending on the situation you may be going through, your preferences, and the tasks you undertake at the moment. It is therefore essential to understand what you can do and take control effectively. You can also understand what you are capable of managing by knowing every of your limitation. You will activate the vagus nerve response accordingly and free yourself from dissociative responses into more manageable ones with such an understanding. Being in your present body or mind helps you to adjust or save yourself from the shutdown mode. It will lead you to live and exist in a lifestyle you knew you could live for a long time.

Chapter 2:
Importance of Polyvagal Theory

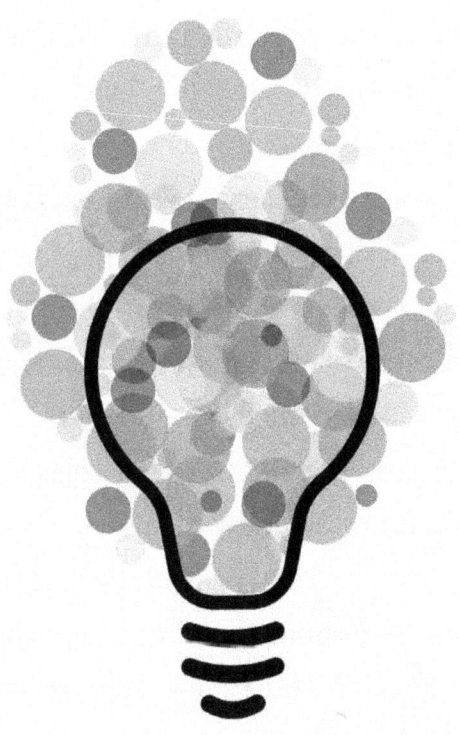

Our approaches and perceptions towards emotions are often complex, ethereal, and troublesome in establishment and implementation. However, it is essential to understand that emotions are external and internal responses to information. In most cases, emotions occur almost suddenly that they catch most people unawares, especially those with no proper understanding of their inner emotional life. Therefore, polyvagal theory comes lively in handy when every person's primal desire to remain alive becomes necessary. It is an essential top-up to our bodies regardless of our confidence in staying alive. As usual, the nervous system is always active in the background dominating other bodily functions. Therefore, it is inarguably true that we can confidently believe in various activities such as the preferable dessert or dinner to take or ways to excel in college. Since it's a crucial system in the body, the nervous system works together with the brain and can control the body's emotional expertise. You can easily understand the nervous system's conjunctive coordination and the vagus nerves through the Polyvagal theory. The theory is beneficial to every individual and tries to determine our reactions and capabilities to develop connections in environments around us. The theory is crucial for psychology experts and therapists because it helps them understand:

- PTSD and trauma
- Attacks and withdrawal in relationships
- How extreme stress results in shutdown or dissociation

- Dealing with mental health
- Learning through body language

Extra benefits of the Polyvagal theory

- Polyvagal theory clinical applications and the vagal nerve tone implemented in psychological and medical analysis.
- Through the vagus nerve mediation, clinical applications in the human fetus result in high variability in vital signs. On the other hand, vital decelerations mediated by the vagus nerve signify distress. More clearly, prolonged withdrawal of the vagal nerve may affect the guts by creating physiological vulnerability to the effect of dorsal vagal nerve management. As a result, victims experience a low heart rate. Before starting this slowing, it is possible to experience tachycardia, whose effects reflect the withdrawal of Ventral vagal management.
- The Polyvagal theory has built human behavior and psychology. Through evolution comes the human nervous system. Therefore, the nervous system gradually developed with special neural and behavioral options through these processes of evolution. The options act on challenges to ensure that the visceral is in a proper physiological state.
- According to the theory, the brain's phyletic origins optimize social and defensive behaviors, domains affected

with syndromes in different persons, and any other psychiatric disorder.
- The Polyvagal theory also connects the autonomic system evolution to experience social behavior, communication, gestures, and emotions. Therefore, the same ensures plausible rationalization of communication, social and emotional behaviors, and other related disorders.
- The theory generates a biological science model that enables us to understand the link between facial expression and visceral state regulation and spontaneous social behavior problems. It also helps us understand how social behavior can regulate the physiological activity.
- The Polyvagal theory tries to suggest an attainable and verifiable mechanism. Some of the difficulties generate a crucial field of most specialty profiles. Concerning the same, psychiatric disorders are the exact deficits common to diagnoses in visceromotor and somatomotor. As a result, the phyletic mechanical phenomenon advances the neural structures responsible for behavior regulation. It is more crucial in cases of social communication behaviors required to interact with others. The phylogenetically modern systems don't majorly provide social communication mechanisms. The systems usually also extend to controlling visceral organs into calm states.
- Through the theory, we acquire a biological science

model crucial justifying how affectional states, social behavior, and positive support may advance health and growth in different ways. As opposed to the health-connected states common to prosocial behavior, removing the new neural system can enhance mobilization behaviors. It is because elongating the periods within which physiological responses occur may result in more damaging outcomes. Therefore, people suffering specific psychiatric disorders related to compromised social behavior may be a diagnostic feature, and that they experience neuroscience states effective for nonsocial and defensive behaviors is verifiable. The phyletic principles underlie most theories related to behavioral and physiological responses concerning psychiatric disorders.

- The theory is crucial in developing a better understanding of safety and danger. It is crucial for supporting proper interaction between bodily primitive experiences and everyone's faces and voices around us.
- The theory explains why a form face or a better tonal voice may adjust or affect the approach we tend to feel. The polyvagal theory also tries to explain the safety and calm we feel after knowing that important people detect and feel our presence around them. It also tries to explain why unemployment may fuel mental collapse or rage reactions.

- The Polyvagal theory advances our perception of why attuning with various persons may drag us out of compromising and fearful states. Therefore, Porges's theory helps us explore a wider aspect of the effects of fight or flight. It thus centers on social relationships as a proper way of understanding traumatic experiences. It suggests new diplomatic approaches to healing through narrowing down to body strengthening to control arousal.

Chapter 3:
The polyvagal Activities and Mind & Body Activities

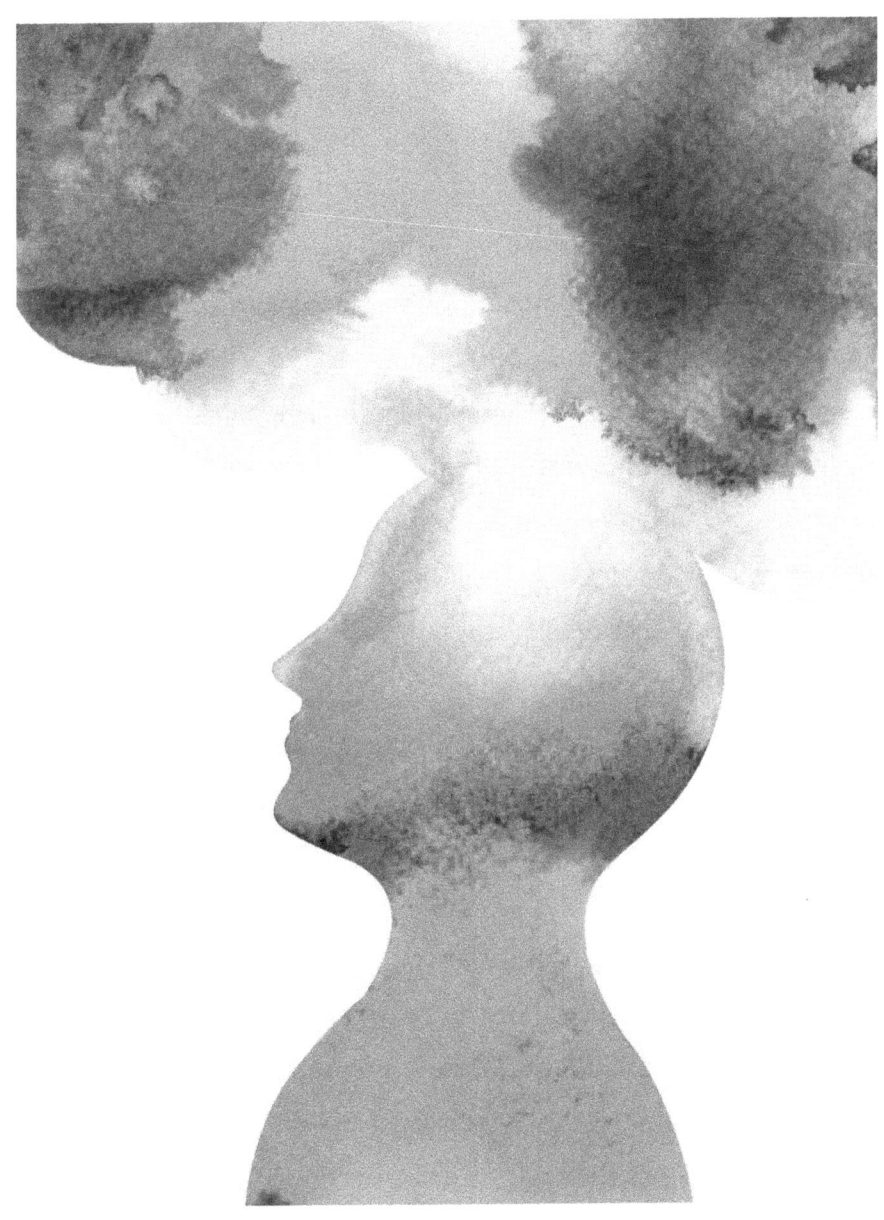

Therapies associated with the mind and body are usually helpful in various instances. They foster adaptive services such as mitigation of harmful effects related to social adversity, allostatic load reduction, and control of self-regulatory resilience and ANS skills across various populations and conditions.

The mind-body therapies suggest forming a source of exercising the neural platforms by affecting the vagal pathways to foster resilience and self-regulation of physiological functions, prosocial behavior, and emotional regulation.

Generation of balanced neural regulation of the autonomic nervous system and relevant immune and the endocrine system occur by the active engagement of the VVC by utilizing specific positions or movements, breathing practices, meditation, or chanting, which affects both bottom-up and top-down processes.

From a polyvagal theory perspective, exercise, mindful, focused attention, and social engagement manipulate physiological state by neural activity. Training demands increased cardiac output through increased sympathetic influences on the heart and a removal of vagal inhibition.

Resilience is kept by supporting more adaptability and flexibility. And by downregulating defensive states in relationship to improve physiological restoration and positive social and psychological states. The Vagus nerve connects the brain to significant systems of the body, including facial muscles, throat, lungs, heart, stomach, and gut.

A healthy vagus nerve helps regulate your sleep pattern, support your digestive system, and calm down your nerves. Regulation of vagal tone is associated with reducing inflammation and a good prognosis in people suffering from chronic illness, autoimmune disorders, anxiety, migraine, and depression.

The parasympathetic influence on the heart is positively associated with engagement coping and various aspects of social well-being. People exposed to interventions that positively affect vagal regulation also experience a high level of positive emotions and more supportive public interactions.

People with long-term, chronic traumatic exposure can lose the capability to perceive whether a situation is safe or trustworthy. In other words, one can feel a location threatening, whereas it is secure. He should learn to override unnecessary defensive reactions of freeze, fight, flight, or faint in such circumstances. In such cases engaging the social nervous system will help to manage vagus nerve disorders.

The social nervous system gets strengthened by repeated practice that myelinated the pathway of the nerve. Engagement of the social nervous system mobilizes the sympathetic nervous system allows to access creativity. Mind-body therapies regulate the vagus nerve and improve resilience through:

- Safe mobilization.
- A safe immobilization.

Initially, it involves the capacity to feel peaceful, connected, and calm. It completes by blending social engagements with mobilization and immobilization. Until the re-establishment of safety develops, it becomes easy to move in and out of different nervous system states over time.

Somatic psychology and mind-body therapies make an individual capable of attending to his thoughts, emotional experiences, breath, and body sensations simultaneously. Some practices involve mindful use of stillness, and others, conscious use of movement.

Mind-body therapies are healing processes that enhance the mind's interactions with bodily functions to create relaxation and increase overall health and well-being. Daily practice is essential to obtain the desired effects. These are effective and safe ways to mitigate the emotional and physical symptoms and improving coping skills in cancer patients.

The Vagus nerve links the heart and muscles of the face, makes it engage in empathic responses. Mind-body interventions involve prayer, cognitive behavioral therapy, imagery, relaxation, biofeedback, hypnosis, meditation, yoga, tai chi, and others.

Acupuncture

It is a traditional therapeutic component of Chinese medicine that involves very thin needles in the presence of electricity, pressure, or heat to stimulate points on the body, improving the flow of balance and internal energy. This mind-body therapy helps to treat chronic pain and symptoms associated with cancer treatment.

Message therapy

This mind-body therapy is effective in alleviating symptoms related to cancer, like anxiety and pain. Oncology guidelines recommend using massage for mood disorders and depression. Message therapy is generally safe and excessively used as a complementary therapy to relieve some symptoms of cancer and other diseases.

Hypnotherapy

In hypnotherapy, a therapist guides the person into a relaxed and focused state and asks him to think about the situations and experiences in positive ways that may help him change the way he behaves or thinks. Hypnotherapy effectively relieves symptoms of sleep problems, generalized anxiety disorders, and physical issues, like irritable bowel syndrome and chronic pain.

Aromatherapy

This is a type of mind-body therapy in which the scent of concentrated oils, called essential oils, improves well-being thoughts. It is a popular therapy used to produce pleasant sensations and to relieve stress.

Biofeedback
Biofeedback involves using auditory or visual feedback to gain control of involuntary bodily functions. It consists of voluntary control of muscle tension, pain perception, blood flow, heart rate, and blood pressure.

The goal of biofeedback is to build insight on how one should physically react to trauma, anxiety, or other mental health issues. So it enables better control of physical symptoms. This mind-body therapy helps relieve symptoms of chronic physical pain associated with addiction, depression and eating disorders, and post-traumatic stress disorder.

Movement therapy
It aims to reconnect your body and mind through movement. This therapy improves the symptoms of those suffering from eating disorders.

Chiropractic Adjustments
This mind-body technique consists of spinal manipulation.

Though this is less common than the others, spinal manipulations or manual therapy combines moving joints, exercise, massage, and physical therapist. It is helpful in lower back pain and headache.

Meditation

In many traditions, it is used for millennia around the globe to improve overall well-being. These practices involve using the mind to regulate breathing, focus on attention, and produce a non-judgmental awareness of feelings and thoughts to achieve internal calm, psychological balance, physical relaxation, and improved coping and vitality.

Tai Chi.

This therapy is an ancient Chinese tradition. It is an exercise program that involves precise body movements, synchronized breathing, and meditation to improve well-being and health.

Qigong

Approximately 5000 years ago, it got developed in China as a form of meditation and exercise. It integrates breathing exercises, muscle relaxation, and body movement to improve emotional, physical, and psychological health.

Yoga

People practice simple breathing exercises, meditation techniques, and physical postures to promote relaxation and health.

Yoga makes the human body have intense vagus activity. In practice, the vagus nerve's engagement during stillness or movement can blend the social nervous system for varying energy levels and health needs.

Breathing maneuvers within yoga may facilitate alterations similarly in the autonomic state with convergent health and psychological consequences. These practices also control our capacity to experience connections beyond public interactions or networks and a more unbounded and universal sense of connection and oneness.

Yoga therapy may alleviate suffering by transforming a person's relationship to the BME phenomenon and catalyzing the emergence of eudaimonic well-being. The eudaimonic condition of the human is a sense of well-being or flourishing that is non-transitory. And it is often connected to a sense of purpose, meaning, or self-realization.

Eudaimonic state of well-being links to health benefits like reduction in perceived loneliness, in response to social adversity mitigation of gene expression improved immune regulation, decreased inflammation, mental flourishing, and reduced all-cause mortality independent of all other variables.

Yoga therapy contributes towards the eudaimonic nervous system to emerge prosocial behaviors and posits that the neuronal platforms supporting social behavior are involved in maintaining restoration, growth, and health.

This model connects the expression of social and emotional behavior and patterns of autonomic regulation. It utilizes an understanding of human behavior, illness, and stress. Like the neural platforms of polyvagal theory, the gunas provide the foundation for the emergence of emotional, behavioral, and physical attributes.

The following steps will help you recover from vagus nerve disorders

Find A Safe Place
First, find a safe place where you think you can practice and explore these mind-body therapies. Find a comfortable position, either seated, standing, or lying down. Look around your place, identify different visual cues that keep you feeling safe. Throughout the practice, repeat to yourself that I am calm, I am connected.

Increase Sensory Awareness
Take some long, deep breaths. Feel the subtle movements created by your breath and sensations of the breath in the body.

Now bring your awareness to the sounds of breathing. Now expand your sensory knowledge to notice some other sensations of your body. Keep repeating the phrase; I am safe; I am calm, I get connected. In case during practice you feel anxiety repeat the first step, remind yourself that you are safe.

Explore Mindful Mobilization

Now, start to explore the intensity of your breath while moving your body. You can stand up into an active yoga posture. You can walk vigorously in your room or around the place. Increase your heart rate, which would enough to notice that your breath gets quick to support your movement. As you move your body, repeat the phrase, I am safe; I am calm; I get connected. At this step, if you feel any anxiety, remind yourself that you are safe.

Explore Mindful Immobilization

In the final step of practice, return to stillness, either seated, standing, or lying down. Make your heart rate slow down. Surrender your bodyweight down towards the earth. To initiate a relaxation response, take deep, long breaths extending your exhale longer than the inhale. Remain still and soften any extra and unnecessary holding in your muscles. As you connect to stillness, repeat the phrase I am safe, I am calm; I get attached. If you experience some distress or anxiety, make yourself remember that you are safe now.

An individual can learn to control activation of the ventral vagal complex with its homeostatic influence on the person and increase the chance to initiate or inhibit the other neural platforms like DVC or SNS when encounters perceived or real stress. As a whole, mind-body therapies can:

- Make the individuals VVC more control able.
- Increase the threshold of tolerance to other neural platforms.
- Alter the response and relationship to DVC and SNS neural pathways that occur on natural fluctuations of BME.
- The person becomes more skilled at moving in and out of these neural pathways.

Mind-body therapies focus on the cultivation of bodily awareness. They involve both proprioception and interoception added with the mindfulness-dependent qualities of non-reactivity, nonjudgement, acceptance, or curiosity to re-appraise stimuli. We support an individual in the process of re-orientation or re-interpretation to such stimuli so that insight may develop and regulation, adaptability and resilience may foster.

Patients are utilizing mind-body therapies for healing report both a shift in their response and experience to negative emotions and feelings and the development of self-regulation skills in dealing with emotional regulations, pain, and re-appraisal of life situations.

Mind-body therapies include yoga therapies, which work by facilitating bidirectional communication. In which contact between mind and body benefit human health and well-being. These practices focus on the integration of:

- ✓ Top-down neurocognitive.
- ✓ Bottom-up neurophysiological mechanisms.

Top-down processes, like regulation of intention and attention, have been shown to decrease the hypothalamic-pituitary axis and psychological stress and sympathetic nervous system activity and modulate inflammation and immune function.

Bottom-up processes get promoted by movement practices and breathing techniques. They influence the nervous system, musculoskeletal, and cardiovascular system function and affect sympathetic nervous system activity and hypophysial-pituitary axis.

The bottom-up and top-down processes employed in mind-body therapies regulate neuroendocrine, autonomic, behavioral, and emotional activation and support an individual's reaction to challenges. Self-regulation is a conscious ability to keep the systems stable to interpret or alter responses to threats or adversity. By decreasing allostatic load, we can shift autonomic states.

It reduces symptoms of adverse conditions, including irritable bowel syndrome, chronic pain, depression, neurodegenerative diseases, and post-traumatic stress disorder. Resilience also benefits mind-body therapies, as it makes the person bounce back in a short time. And adopts in reaction to adverse and stressful circumstances, the psychophysiological resources are conserved. High resilience is related to quick cardiovascular recovery after subjective emotional experiences.

If you perceived less stress, you would have excellent recovery from trauma and illness and better manage chronic pain and dementia. An imbalance of the autonomic nervous system leads to compromised resilience through measures of vagal regulation. Mind-body therapies like yoga correlate with both improvements in vagal management and psychological resilience.

Chapter 4:
The Impact of Nervous System on Our Bodies

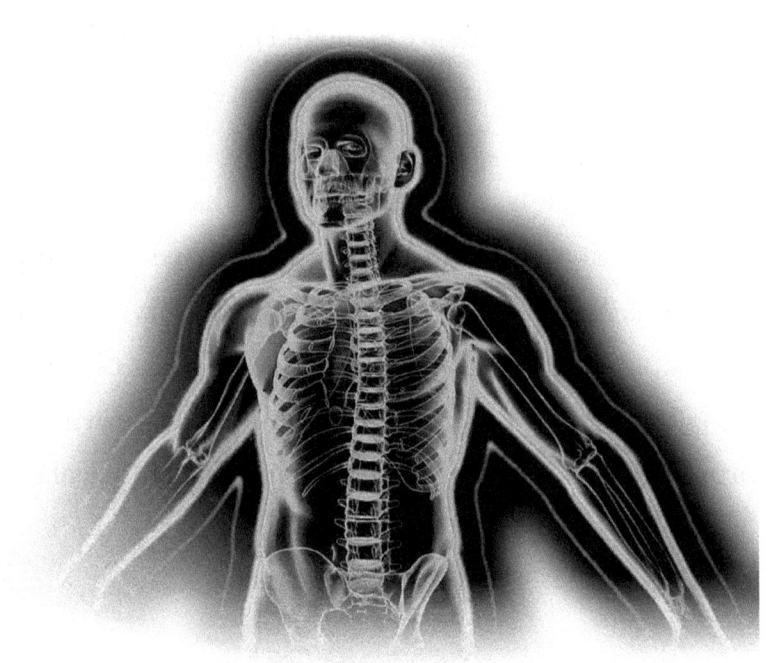

At times, we often experience anxiety issues, stress, and depression. We hope for brighter days, hoping that everything will be back in place and have a peaceful life.

According to research, some of the causes of death are anxiety, depression, and feelings of boredom and loneliness. The world has become one of survival of the fittest. People wake up in the morning with many to-do-s lined up for the day that, in most cases, consume the moments meant for resting and self-reflection.

We are used to working very early in the morning and getting back home later in the evening. Even after work, a person can have some activities to attend to before reaching home.

For example, students in post-secondary and high-school usually have many things to work upon. There are assignments, note-taking, revising, and at the same time, they have to attend to other daily duties at home. Apart from that, they need to socialize with family and friends.

Although technology has offered numerous benefits to society and the ease with which it helps us carry out our work, it has made other things more complex.

We behold celebrities' glamorous lifestyles, and we feel that our lives are like a puzzle that's missing pieces. We go through social media and see friends and strangers alike having the time of

their lives while we lay in bed, thinking of what to squeeze out for a meal. We often tend to ignore it, but accumulated depressive feelings combined with everyday stress can leave us feeling that there is something wrong with our lives when there isn't.
If you want to improve in a given situation, start by accepting the situation and understanding it.

Understanding the problem helps you adjust your attitude toward certain situations and solve the problem appropriately. In this case, the source is one of your body systems. That is why this book exploits more on the Nervous system, which is a vital system in our bodies.

Understanding the Autonomic Nervous System?

At some point, you have heard of the word nervous system. It is a significant part of the body responsible for coordinating all the body's functions and activities by sending signals when passing information from one part of the body to the other. The nerve cell is the special cell that enables this process to be successful.

The nervous system is divided into two vital sections:
The autonomic nervous system (ANS).
The ANS is also known as the vegetative nervous system. It is the part of the peripheral nervous system whose purpose is to

control internal organs such as lungs, glands, blood vessels, genitals, blood vessels, heart, smooth muscles, etc. This system carries out activities in the body unconsciously or without thought, such as respiration, heart rate, urination, digestion, and sexual arousal. It is also in charge of the fight-flight-freeze response. The intellectual Walter Cannon first discovered this theory.

The hypothalamus found in the brain controls all the functions of ANS. For instance, the hypothalamus controls automatic body activities like breathing, heartbeat, and reflexes such as sneezing, vomiting, and coughing.

These functions are still subdivided into different areas and linked to subsystems of the ANS. The hypothalamus, which is located just a bit above the brain stem, integrates these autonomic functions. This system is one of the most important systems in the human body, as any disorder of this system may be progressive or irreversible and can affect the entire body.

The ANS is further divided into three sub-groups. There is the parasympathetic nervous system, the sympathetic nervous, and the enteric nervous system. However, the enteric nervous system hasn't yet been globally recognized as part of the ANS, and some educative materials do not include it. Therefore, we will highlight more on the sympathetic nervous and the parasympathetic nervous system.

- **The Parasympathetic Nervous System**

The parasympathetic nervous system regulates the unconscious activities when the body is at rest, often after eating. In contrast, the autonomic nervous system regulates the unconscious actions of the body. These activities include salivation, lacrimation (flow of tears), sexual arousal, digestion, urination, defecation, among others. They are often known as 'feed and breed' or 'rest and digest' activities. The function of the PSNS complements that of the sympathetic nervous system, which regulates fight-flight-freeze responses.

Parasympathetic nerves have a craniosacral outflow (they exit the CNS from the brain stem or the sacral region of the spine), compared to the sympathetic system with a thoracolumbar outflow.

- **The Sympathetic Nervous System**

At some point, every person has experienced some fears. Some fears can be extreme, while others are mild. What matters is that we all understand and know what it takes to experience fear.

The way you respond to fear is known as the fight-flight-freeze response (or acute stress response). This response is controlled and managed by the sympathetic nervous system. It is usually active at a low level to regulate homeostasis, which is equilibrium and harmony in the body.

But then, how does it work?

Sympathetic nerves begin in the central nervous system in the spine sections known as the thoracic spine and the lumbar spine. It is often known as the thoracolumbar outflow because the axons or ends of these cells exit the spine here and communicate or synapse with either sympathetic ganglion cells or specialized cells in the kidneys and the adrenal glands found at the top of the kidneys.

Sympathetic neurons emit neurotransmitters or chemicals called epinephrine and norepinephrine (also known as adrenaline and noradrenaline). Adrenaline jumpstarts the body into action, with effects such as increased heart rate, diverting blood flow from the organs toward the skeletal muscles, dilating pupils, and increasing sweating, for example.

Sympathetic nerves that connect to the kidneys release a chemical called dopamine. Dopamine can be turned into norepinephrine (noradrenaline) in the adrenal glands if the body signals for it. Sympathetic nerves connected to chromaffin cells in the adrenal glands produce substantial epinephrine (adrenaline) from norepinephrine). Both epinephrine and norepinephrine result in responses that ready the body for action under stress.

Why is this system known as the 'sympathetic' nervous system, of all things? History has it that this name stems from the idea of sympathy. Sympathy is the perception of someone's or something's distress and reacting accordingly, so it was thought of in the sense of having a connection between parts or people.

The Central Nervous System

The CNS- central nervous system and the PNS-peripheral nervous system. The CNS is made up of the brain and spinal cord, the importance of which is obvious. The brain controls all body functions, including movement, awareness, thought, speech, memory, and much more. The spinal cord is linked to a portion of the brain called the brainstem, where it sends messages from the brain to the peripheral nerves and vice versa, and it also plays a vital role in body positioning.

The peripheral nervous system can be said to oversee all activities which take place in the body apart from the brain and spinal cord, or the CNS. Its role is to ensure that the various body parts are communicating well and working in harmony. When communication is at its peak, we react appropriately to the various stimuli we sense from the environment.

You are probably asking yourself where the autonomic nervous system fits into all of this.

The peripheral nervous system is divided into two parts:
the SNS-somatic nervous system and the ANS -autonomic nervous system

The word 'somatic' is derived from the Greek word 'soma,' which means 'body.' This implies that the somatic nervous system is responsible for sending and receiving motor and sensory information either to or from the CNS. It is also a major player involuntary movement. To this effect, this system consists of two major types of neurons —sensory and motor neurons— which carry information from the body to the brain and spinal cord and from the brain and spinal cord to the body, respectively. It is their actions that result in response to physical stimuli.

So, what is the structure of this system?

The nerves in this system are autonomic, and their supply primarily stems from these three sources: the cranial nerves, the vagus nerve, and the pelvic splanchnic nerves.

Parasympathetic nerves (a special type of cranial nerve) stem from particular nuclei (groups of nerve cells in the CNS) and form a synapse at any of the four parasympathetic ganglia (groups of nerve cells outside the CNS or in the PNS). From there, these nerves reach their target tissues through trigeminal nerves (nerves that are responsible for motor and sensory functions). Another type of cranial nerve is called the oculomotor nerve, which regulates most eye-related parasympathetic functions.

The vagus nerve originates in the lower half of the brain stem, which is connected to the spinal cord (known as the brain stem medulla). The term 'vagus nerve' originates from the Latin word 'vagus,' which means 'wandering.' This is appropriate considering that this nerve controls many target tissues. However, the vagus nerve is quite unusual because it doesn't follow the trigeminal nerve path to reach its destination (the target tissues). This nerve is also very difficult to trace because it is virtually everywhere in the thorax and abdomen. Several parasympathetic nerves leave the vagus nerve as they enter the thorax, such as the laryngeal and cardiac nerves. The organs affected by the abdomen's parasympathetic nerves include the pancreas, kidney, and gall bladder.

The pelvic splanchnic nerves exit the spine through the sacral region. They contribute immensely to the supply of nerves to the genital and pelvic organs. They regulate urinary excretion, the sensation of pain, and sexual functions like penis erection.

Remember when it was stated that the parasympathetic nervous system has a cranio-sacral outflow? The pelvic splanchnic nerves are an important sacral component of the PSNS. It is equivalent to the sacral splanchnic nerves that emerge from the sympathetic trunk in the SNS.

Parasympathetic nerves produce the neurotransmitter acetylcholine, which the target organs receive, which response by stimulating parasympathetic activities.

Relationship Between the Sympathetic and Parasympathetic Nervous Systems

The interesting thing about the autonomic nervous system's sympathetic and parasympathetic components is that they work opposite each other. First, the SNS controls actions that require quick and immediate response while the PSNS controls slower or delayed activities. Furthermore, the SNS speeds up the body processes, for example, increasing the heart rate when faced with imminent danger. The PSNS, on the other hand, calms the body, for example, reducing heart rate.

Muscles stimulated by the SNS contract while those stimulated by the PSNS relax. The SNS releases adrenaline while the PSNS has no connection with the adrenal gland. The same goes for glycogen conversion; the SNS transforms glycogen into glucose for muscle energy. The bronchial tubes constrict when influenced by the PSNS but dilate under the influence of the SNS. There is an increase in urinary output when the PSNS is active, while the opposite happens with SNS activity. The neurons in the PSNS are cholinergic (produce and receive acetylcholine), while in the SNS, neurons are adrenergic (produce and receive norepinephrine/epinephrine).

The Enteric Nervous System (ENS)

Otherwise known as the intrinsic nervous system, the ENS is one of the systems in the ANS. Its neurons' system in the lining of the gastrointestinal tract regulates the GI tract activities from the esophagus down to the anus. One powerful thing about this system is that it can work without the sympathetic and parasympathetic systems but may be affected by them. The ENS, also more trendily known as the gut, is sometimes referred to as the second brain.

This system operates without the brain and the spinal cord but needs the supply of nerves from the autonomic nervous system through the prevertebral ganglia and vagus nerve. However, research has shown that the enteric nervous system can function even with a severed vagus nerve. The neurons from this system not only secrete enzymes from the gastrointestinal tract but also regulate motor functions.

The ENS contains over 500 million neurons. There are millions of neurons in the spinal cord alone. These neurons interact via neurotransmitters that are almost the same as those used in the CNS, and they include dopamine, serotonin, and acetylcholine.

The Function of the Autonomic Nervous System in the Body

Recall that the autonomic nervous system is a division of the peripheral nervous system, which is a division of the nervous system as a whole. The ANS is responsible for regulating functions that are carried out without conscious effort. It was then stated that the ANS has two divisions—the sympathetic nervous system (SNS) and the parasympathetic nervous system (PSNS). Therefore, it would be fitting to say that the ANS functions are the functions of the individual divisions. The SNS takes care of fight-or-flight responses. The PSNS takes care of the actions the body undertakes at rest, especially after eating. The ENS takes care of the activities of the gastrointestinal tract.

So, what exactly are the functions of these systems?

Functions of the Sympathetic Nervous System

It dilates the bronchioles of the lungs by spreading epinephrine continuously, thereby improving oxygen exchange.

It relaxes the ciliary muscles in the eye linked to the lens and dilates pupils, thereby allowing more light to penetrate the eye.

It regulates homeostasis. This function does not just apply to human beings but all living organisms. The fibers in this system supply nerves to the tissues of almost every organ in the body. This process regulates diverse functions like blood flow, urinary control, pupil dilation and constriction, body temperature, blood sugar levels, pH, etc.

-It activates an organism

-It regulates the fight-or-flight response, sometimes called fight-flight-freeze response or the sympathoadrenal response (derived from the words' sympathetic' and 'adrenal medulla'). This is one of the most vital functions of the SNS. It controls the hormonal and neuronal stress response. The preganglionic fibers in the system activate epinephrine release (adrenaline) in great quantities, acting directly on the cardiovascular system. When activated, the SNS or fight-or-flight response:

- ✓ Boosts blood flow to the lungs and skeletal muscles.
- ✓ Constricts blood vessels, especially those in the kidney and skin. This happens when the adrenergic receptors are activated by norepinephrine that is released by postganglionic neurons. This also causes a redirection of blood flow from the skin and gastrointestinal tract.
- ✓ It prevents peristalsis, thereby preventing digestion.
- ✓ Allows the heart's coronary vessels to widen or relax, especially the ones in large arteries, large veins, and smaller arterioles.

-It gets the body ready for action, especially in life-threatening situations. For instance, the SNS prepares your body in the morning before waking up by increasing its outflow spontaneously.

-It stimulates sweat excretion in sweat glands.

-It increases heart rate. The contribution of both the sympathetic and parasympathetic nervous systems to the sinoatrial node regulates heart rate. Note that heart rate is different from heart rhythm. Heart rate is the number of times the heart beats per second, while the heart rhythm is the heartbeats pattern. When the heart rate is increased, blood flow to the heart and active skeletal muscles is improved.

-It prevents tumescence or swelling. Penis tumescence is commonly known as penis erection, which entails blood filling the penis in preparation for sexual activity. When faced with life-threatening situations, the SNS prevents this from occurring.

-It constricts all intestinal and urinary sphincters.

Functions of the Parasympathetic Nervous System

Recall that the parasympathetic nervous system functions directly opposite to the sympathetic nervous system. The PSNS:

-Lowers the heart rate by producing acetylcholine, contrary to the sympathetic nervous system, which increases heart rate by producing epinephrine and norepinephrine (or adrenaline and noradrenaline).

-Increases blood flow by relaxing or widening blood vessels that are linked to the gastrointestinal tract.

Enhances near vision by contracting the pupil and constricting the ciliary muscles in the eye. This is the opposite of what the SNS does, which is to enhance far vision.

-Aids sexual activity. The nerves in this system help to erect the genital tissues through the pelvic splanchnic nerves. When a man is about to ejaculate, the sympathetic system causes the internal pelvic sphincter to close and the urethral muscle to undergo peristalsis. Likewise, the parasympathetic system causes peristalsis to occur in the urethral muscle, and the bulbospongiosus muscles are contracted by the pudendal nerve to violently discharge the semen. The penis becomes flaccid again afterward.

-Improves absorption of nutrients by enhancing the secretion of saliva and the rate of peristalsis.

Reduces the diameter of the bronchioles when the body needs less oxygen.

Functions of the Enteric Nervous System

The ENS (also known as the second brain) has its unique function since it is the nervous system that coordinates the gastrointestinal system's processes. The ENS:

-Acts as a neuron integrating unit. This system is called the second brain primarily because it can exist on its own. It interacts with the CNS through the prevertebral ganglia and the vagus nerve, but it can still function autonomously when the vagus nerve is severed.

Because this system comprises several kinds of neurons (neurons that both send and receive signals), it can stand in for the CNS input as an integrating unit. These neurons act on chemical and mechanical conditions.

-Controls GI tract secretions. Gastrointestinal enzymes are controlled by cholinergic neurons that are located on the walls of the digestive tract.

Chapter 5:
Dealing with Autism and Mental Stress

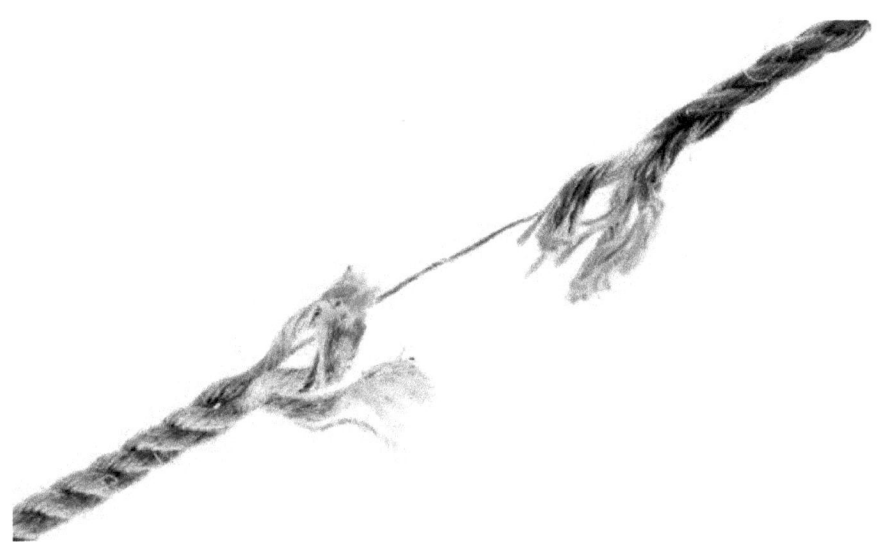

Autism is among the diseases that experts research more often. People who have Autism have difficulty differentiating general ideas and thoughts. Showing the impact of Autism on the Brain and heart is a point that has been still being Research, and there are new researches that have been putting forward to it. Autism is not a psychological disorder. It can be termed as a behavioral or developmental disability because people suffering from Autism have difficulty communicating and having social interactions. They also have many challenges in their behavior and upbringing because people who suffer from Autism are uncategorized differently from normal people who don't suffer from Autism. Their brain function is quite complex, and why different from people who are not suffering from the problems of people with Autism is very challenging. They might need more help in a different part of life than those who are not suffering from autism. People who are suffering from Autism have certain behavior patterns that are repetitive and then not changed in their daily activities. They have difficulty paying attention and react to different things differently, and the signs that are often started from early childhood. It becomes more prominent while the child is going into higher education. The child has difficulty in school, which is when a child at the school with Autism starts to be reported. A child reacts differently to certain behavior and Society and color. Their child may be not Show interest in every other thing. They might not have the same perception of things as other people because their brains are a complex part of the change. They have difficulty in relating to other people; that's why they don't interrupt because they have difficulty in understanding what they are trying to say no matter how hard it is, and they always like isolating them because they find it pretty awkward to have eye contact and they have difficulty in doing so.

Even after having so many cases of Autism, there is no proper way of testing and of knowing the child is autistic because there is no medical test for it to diagnose.

The only diagnosis that can be made is on the child's behavior and development, and it can be detected at an early age of 11. On the other hand, in adults, people have the fun of people having more acceptance and more awareness of this because of the research and more movies and books written on it.

The heart: Autistic kids or adults are more prone to having a disease than a person who is not autistic, which is the nervous system controlling a heart rate. It might be a little offbeat or slightly different in autistic people because people who are having Autism have a steady variable that is constant. It hardly varies in frequency, which is because of the autonomic nervous system. It is the nerves of sensory nerves that control the Heartbeat and the human body.

In autistic people, it's slightly off for them that is why the interval of Heartbeat vary even if the people are not doing anything for normal people but for people with Autism, no matter the doing anything of the doing Cardio exercise if they are running they would always have a constant heart rate, or it would be an interesting way because with it later on it becomes like a processing problem, so they tend to have more cognitive hard diseases as compared to a normal person. There is a reduced heart rate or a resting heart rate in people who have autism. many researchers happened stating that people who have heart disease is linked to Autism of people, which might also have a connection, but the fact is that people who have Autism might have been an increased rate of having a heart disease

The Brain: A brain is like a circuit in everybody's body to know if there is any impact of Autism on the Brain. Autistic people, according to researchers that had happened to understand the circuit of the human brain, which is a complex circuit, and they wanted to see if there is a way on which the brain reacts in autistic people. Difficulty in switching up in processes and understanding different judgments it gets hard for them to come up with any sort of answer. in a very simple or Complex situation as compared to a normal person's brain. It might surprise many people that the people who have Autism have a very symmetrical brain because, in neurological or psychological disorders, the brain's hemisphere starts to differ from each other. They are not very alike, but in Autism, they seem to reflect the right and left for synthetic reflection of each other because they are so alike. Despite the reaction to certain stimuli differently because certain challenges of life become more challenging for them, they have difficulty making new friends in socializing. They have difficulty communicating with people around them. It is mainly the process of stimuli. They have variations in behavior and impact because of the neurological difference in the head that is caused by the brain. The brain becomes less rewarding for social motivation as compared to the children who don't have Autism. what happens if that children who suffer from Autism have difficulty in social interaction? They don't like socializing. they don't like having contact with different people, and it is more common in younger children. The system in an autistic child of the brain works very differently because they would find different interests more rewarding than the normal ones, so they differ from normal children even though it is not enough normality. It is not such a big difference between is Autism should be normalized, and the kids are not abnormal because it is not an abnormality in a child how it can also be taken as a neurological thing. it is not abnormal for the child. It can be declared abnormal after this the sensor symptoms that come because of the brain's neurons. it is said that because Autism and its effect on the brain are so that they have too much brain activity going on, they find it difficult to react to certain things. For example, if a child is concentrating in a completely autistic child might find it difficult to concentrate or a lot of activities going in their mind because they have an overly intense brain.

The brain they have is fluctuated and consists of so many activities going on in one situation that they find it hard to think and hide and difficulty concentrating. That is why it is said that autistic children have difficulty in focus. The difficulty in focusing is not because the brain does not work that way; it is because the brain is more intense. a brain has the capability of multitasking because with it goes overboard and the lack in certain situations and children with Autism might feel things more as compared to a normal child does not have because in autism working this way on the brain that if there is any noise processed in the brain define it too loud. Colors didn't find it more appealing. it is a way that the sensory nerves in the brain have been caught up. they are too sensitive to sharp colors or loud noises because of the sensory stimulation caused by Autism in the brain. They react strongly to certain sensations that might be normal for the children; that is why sensory symptoms such as shouting or certain Complex sentences they have are more responsive. parents are more concerned about this part of the child; however, Autism leads to Responsibility in the brain, which is how they react. based on what they think might be the end, not because of the People's attention because of which the brain needs more attention, and it also gives out more attention to certain areas where no attention is needed at all. They focus on areas that do not need too much attention, and they have difficulty in memory. They have difficulty in functioning and planning because these things happening higher in the brain function happened. They also have social cognition, and children with Autism also have more activity in the brain than other people, and they also have difficulty portraying anything emotionally. Autism causes overactivity of things, and the preferred cortex also causes many other sensory reactions, but there are more of those with Autism. autistic children are not a curse to society. There is more to the Brain; autistic children may notice very small details because they observe more in silence, but they are very observant. They observe things more personally and have an amazing memory. If they are told one thing, they might remember it even after 25-30 years because that is how the brain reacts. They would always remember important details and will always know every single small or big detail because the brain works that way.

The symptoms and effects of autism on the life of children

It is a condition identified with mental health that impacts how an individual sees and associates with others, messing up social cooperation and correspondence. The confusion additionally incorporates restricted and tedious examples of conduct. Mental imbalance range issue starts in youth and the long run, causes problems working in the public arena — socially, in school and grinding away. Regularly youngsters show side effects of mental imbalance inside the first year. Few kids seem to grow typically in the primary year and afterward experience a time of relapse somewhere in the range of 18 and two years old enough when they create mental imbalance side effects.

While there is no solution for autism spectrum disorder (ASD), escalated, early treatment can significantly affect numerous kids' lives. ASD is unique in various individuals. It's a developmental handicap that influences how individuals impart, carry on, or associate with others. There's no single reason for it, and indications can be extraordinarily severe or mellow. A few kids on the spectrum begin giving indications as youthful as a couple of months old. Others appear to have an ordinary improvement for the initial scarcely any months or long periods of their lives, and afterward, they begin demonstrating manifestations. Up to half of the guardians of youngsters with ASD saw issues when their kid arrived at a year, and somewhere in the range of 80% and 90% saw problems by two years. Youngsters with ASD will have indications for the duration of their lives, yet it's feasible for them to show signs of improvement as they get more seasoned.

The spectrum of autism is extremely wide. A few people may have genuinely observable issues, and others may not. The repeating theme is contrasts in social abilities, correspondence, and conduct contrasted and individuals who aren't on the range.

Symptoms

Social Skills:
A baby with ASD will some hard memories associating with others. Issues with social aptitudes are the most ordinary signs. He may look to have intimate connections but does not know how to build them.

If your child is on the main spectrum, he may give some social manifestations when he's 8 to 10 months old. These may incorporate any of the accompanyings:

- ✓ He can't react to his name from his first birthday celebration.
- ✓ Playing, sharing, or conversing with others doesn't intrigue him.
- ✓ He likes to be distant from everyone else.
- ✓ He stays away from or rejects physical contact.
- ✓ He stays away from the eye to eye connection.
- ✓ When he's vexed, he doesn't prefer to be improved.
- ✓ He doesn't get emotions - his own or others'.
- ✓ He may not widen his arms to be gotten or guided with strolling.

Communication

Most have a few issues, including these:
- ✓ Delayed discourse and language aptitudes

- ✓ Flat, automated talking voice, or tiresome sound
- ✓ Echolalia (rehashing the same expression again and again)
- ✓ Problems with pronouns (speaking "you" rather than "I," for instance)
- ✓ Not using or once in a while utilizing regular motions (pointing or waving), and also not giving reactions to them
- ✓ Inability to stay on the point when talking or responding to questions
- ✓ Not perceiving mockery or kidding

Behaviors

- ✓ Kids with ASD additionally act in manners that appear to be irregular or have interests that aren't regular. Instances of this can include:
- ✓ Repetitive activities like hand-fluttering, shaking, bouncing, or whirling
- ✓ Constant moving (pacing) and "hyper" conduct
- ✓ Fixations on specific exercises or articles
- ✓ Specific schedules or ceremonies (and getting resentful when a routine is changed, even somewhat)
- ✓ Extreme affectability to contact, light, and sound
- ✓ Not participating in "pretend" play or mimicking others' activities
- ✓ Fussy dietary routines
- ✓ Loss of coordination, ungainliness

- ✓ Impulsiveness (as acting without deduction)
- ✓ Aggressive behavior, both with self as well as other people
- ✓ Short ability to focus

Spotting Signs and Symptoms

The previous treatment for mental imbalance range issues starts, the more like it is to be viable. That is the reason realizing how to distinguish the signs and indications is so significant. Make a meeting with your kid's pediatrician if he doesn't meet these particular formative achievements, or if he meets yet loses them later on:

- ✓ Smiles by a half-year
- ✓ Imitates outward appearances or sounds by nine months
- ✓ Coos or chatters by a year
- ✓ Gestures (focuses or waves) from 14 months as well
- ✓ Speaks with same words by 16 months and utilizations expressions of two words or more by two years
- ✓ Plays imagine or "pretend" by year and a half

As they develop, a few youngsters with mental imbalance range issues become progressively drawn in with others and show less unsettling influences in conduct. A few, as a rule, those with the least severe matters, in the end, may lead typical or close ordinary lives. Nonetheless, others keep on experiencing issues with language or social abilities, and the teenage years can bring more regrettable conduct and enthusiastic issues.

Effects of Autism

It is a formative issue described by disabilities in social correspondence and correspondence and the nearness of confined or dull exercises. The beginning of chemical imbalance is before the age of three. The etiology of mental imbalance is natural; however, no single pathologic occasion has been recognized as exceptionally or all around related to the turmoil. The conclusion of mental imbalance can be made precisely at two years old, with social and correspondence disabilities introducing essential impairments. Treatments specific to a chemical imbalance and start at young ages have been found to add noteworthy gains in psychological, social, and language functioning. Thus, a few specific expert practice parameters underline the significance of both early recognizable proof and early mediation in advancing increasingly positive results for youngsters with autism.

Current commonness gauges propose that around three to five youngsters for each 1,000 are influenced with a chemical imbalance range disorder. These appraisals are higher for first-degree family members; the repeat pace of chemical imbalance in kin has been accounted for somewhere in the range of 2% and 8%.13 Individuals with mental imbalance length the whole scope of psychological capacity, with the greater part is working in mental impediment. A considerable extent is working inside the normal to the better-than-expected scope of knowledge.

Kids with mental imbalance may not arrive at indistinguishable formative achievements from their friends, or they may show a loss of social or language aptitudes recently created. For example, a 3-year-old without mental imbalance may show enthusiasm for basic rounds of pretend. A 5-year-old without mental imbalance may appreciate participating in exercises with other youngsters. A youngster with mental imbalance may experience difficulty communicating with others or abhorrence it out and out. Kids with autism may likewise participate in monotonous practices, experience issues resting, or impulsively eat nonfood things. They may think that it's difficult to flourish without an organized domain or predictable daily practice. If your minor has autism, you may need to work intimately with their educators to guarantee they prevail in the study hall. Numerous assets are accessible to assist kids with autism, just as their friends and family. It is a nonexclusive term that portrays a scope of issues identifying with mental health. There will be impacts on how a kid with mental imbalance will learn and create. In any case, what are these obstructions, and would they be able to be survived? Autism impacts youngsters and grown-ups from numerous points of view, but huge numbers of the issues can be survived, or with little changes to how things are done, kids and grown-ups can get to learning. With autism courses featuring regular issues and potential arrangements, correspondence, social association, and dreary practices won't obstruct education and advancement.

All kids figure out how to impart such that feels good to them; however, for some kids determined to have autism, their discourse can be deferred. Focusing just on creating jargon is just a piece of the arrangements. Empowering different correspondence methods, for example, driving, pointing, pictures, and marking, can assist understudies with autism to get to learning. Gesture-based communication is generally utilized with youngsters and grown-ups who cannot hear; however, there is research to propose that instructing kids with autism gesture-based communication can profit them. Now and again, catchphrases are marked and comprehended by others as this can forestall kids become baffled that nobody appears to get them. Watchword Sign, once known as Makaton, is demonstrating useful and an essential device in helping kids get to learning such that they feel great. But, some of the time, it isn't simply getting to learning with correspondence that is the issue. Numerous kids with mental imbalance discover following bearings and understanding what is being asked of them troublesome. The arrangement is about how educators and instructing collaborators associate with kids. Educators and care staff, alongside guardians, should change how they give guidance – would it be that you are requesting that the youngster do. There are numerous different methods for connecting and speaking with understudies with autism, which are discussed in detail in different autism courses.

A significant piece of a kid's advancement is learning through play and associating with others. However, a few kids with Autistic Spectrum Disorder (ASD) can locate this troublesome. For instance, an innovative game can be hard for a youngster on the spectrum with an exacting comprehension of the world. But, inside instruction, we frequently request that understudies 'envision' being another person from a better place or time. There must be an agreeing line that there are a few pieces of conduct displayed by kids with autism that we can't change. Furthermore, as opposed to concentrating on transform, we ought to urge them to learn and investigate the world that sounds good to them.

A few youngsters don't need social connections. This way, a sheltered situation for them to accomplish something tranquil, for example, read or play all alone, isn't an independent arrangement; however, it permits them to see the world from a protected spot.

A few kids with autism can show monotonous conduct that can be a critical hindrance to attempting new things, just as to their learning. It can prompt limited interests and in this manner, asking them to adequately stretch out is troublesome. The answer for some instructors and collaborators is to stop or limit access to the fixation. Yet, consider this, for some youngsters, this monotonous conduct is what keeps them quiet. The tearing of paper, tapping their hands together, a fixation on the illustrious family, etc., are, for the most part, models showed by certain kids. Removing it prompts problematic passionate upheaval, which in itself is a hindrance to learning. Rather, we should hope to coordinate their fixation here. For example, there is a learning procedure for papier mache for a youngster who tears paper or utilizing exploration of the regal family as an artistic exercise. Timetabling in 'extra time' for the understudy to enjoy this fixation has also resulted in a successful method for limiting disturbance and keeping them quiet. Kids are recognized as sitting at various focuses on the spectrum of autism; thus, what works for one kid to assist them with getting to learning may not be so fruitful with another. This is also the essence of empowering understudies to get to training: learning exercises should be formed to the kid's need and not the reverse way around. Youngsters with chemical imbalance may locate those specific activities to reduce dissatisfaction and advance by and large prosperity. Any kind of activity that your kid appreciates can be valuable. Strolling and having a fabulous time in the play area are both perfect.

Mental Stress and Polyvagal Theory

The Polyvagal Theory gives a few experiences into the ingenious idea of physiological state. To start with, the Polyvagal Theory emphasizes that physiological states support various types of conduct. For instance, a physiological state, represented by a vagus nerve withdrawal, would support fight and flight activation practices. Conversely, a physiological state, described by prolonged vagal impact (through pathways beginning in the nucleus ambiguous) on the heart, would strengthen unrestrained social commitment practices.

Second, the Polyvagal theory emphasizes the practical and assisting connections between neural control of the face's striated muscles and the viscera's smooth muscles. Third, the Polyvagal Theory proposes a system, neuroception, to trigger or to restrict defense methodologies. Neuroception, as a procedure, decides if definite highlights in nature inspire specific physiological states that would reinforce either fight \flight or social commitment practices. Neuroception may include zones of the transient cortex that release organic development and eminent social connections' aptitude.

The Polyvagal Theory stresses the neurophysiological and neuroanatomical differentiation between two parts of the vagus nerve. And it suggests that each branch has different, versatile behavioral procedures. The theory tells three phylogenetic phases of the development of the autonomic sensory system of living beings. Each stage is related to a particular autonomic subsystem or circuit held and communicated in adult individuals.

These autonomic subsystems are phylogenetically requested and typically connected to social communication (e.g., facial appearance, vocalization, listening), mobilization (e.g., fight-flight behavior) immobilization.

The social communication framework (i.e., Social Engagement System) depends upon the myelinated vagus's activities, which serves to encourage calm behavioral states by repressing the sympathetic impacts to the heart and depressing the HPA center.

The mobilization framework is dependent on the working of the sympathetic neural system. The phylogenetic segment, the immobilization framework, relies on the unmyelinated or "vegetative" vagus imparted to most vertebrates. With expanded neural multifaceted nature because of phylogenetic development, the individual's conduct and ability to react when stressed is enhanced. The three circuits can be conceptualized as powerful, giving versatile reactions to safe, dangerous, or hazardous events and contexts.

Concerning stress, these subdivisions respond not just to the instant safety or risk in their condition yet to an association between the quick situation and a feeling of activating action dependent on previous events. Subsequently, suppose somebody is experiencing an event in adulthood where they did not have a sense of security. In that case, a situation in their current life may resonate with such an experience. And this individual may become rude and distant as the nervous system automatically turns itself off to endure the stress.

Every one of us suffers from stress in our lives regardless of whether it was an event that causes so much pain and fear and left us helpless. Whether it was a sequence of events that fears us, confuses us, or makes us feel unsafe, any of these experiences can stay in the nervous system for a long time and cause pain and terror to us.

Reactions inside ones' brain might be visible or inconspicuous, which can be mistaken for help. Individual, friend, or relative, if they see the sufferer's internal system is shutting down, they should come forward and offer their help to the individual. They may think the individual responds rudely and outrageously to the people. By applying some cognitive techniques, one can be helped out of the trauma one is facing. Observing that the reaction to the condition is real and substantial, dependent on the individual's neuroception, an advisor or specialist must make the sufferer overcome his stress. Understanding that there is no place for blunders and mistakes, the reaction is certainly not voluntarily made, not thinking about the response clearly and providing safety.

As humans, we have few basic reactions to push, including fight, flight, freeze, offer, and add. Earlier it was reorganized to fight/flight or rest/review, and it is 'freeze' that is more current and uses the Polyvagal Theory. The freeze (or blackout) response is the sensory system playing dead by bringing down the pulse rate, lessening the capacity to hear, reducing the ability to process sounds and words, and possibly influence memory following the occasion, as instances of what it looks like.

Note that freeze response, and the entirety of the stress reactions, are called up not only in dangerous times. They can likewise be assumed as dangerous events. Furthermore, if a person is introduced to a stressful event or any dangerous event, a person might get a panic attack or consider it a higher risk than before. Regardless of whether the body reads the threat effectively, the body is doing and can be expected with the information it needs to protect you and your life.

We are bio-psycho-social animals, and the reaction of our body towards it is versatile. Whatever your stress response is, it is normal. We are all individuals, and our body is doing effective work to make us healthy and is responsible for keeping us alive. Fabulously, your reaction can be refreshed with new information. This is a dynamic property of human beings. There are explicit activities that can support emotional and body knowledge, so the results are present conditions as different to a memory of a past event, including:

- Create body mindfulness and relieve the stress
- Figure out how to self-manage using polyvagal theory
- Get protected
- Find calming social engagement eye contacts, smile, whispering.
- Take deep breaths and try breathing exercises to ensure safety.

The core of relational neurobiology has demonstrated we are supported to react to our environment, particularly individuals, in the development and improvement, and maybe healing, of our sensory systems. We are social animals and can change and adapt ourselves accordingly.

Chapter 6:
Trauma Experiences and Polyvagal Theory

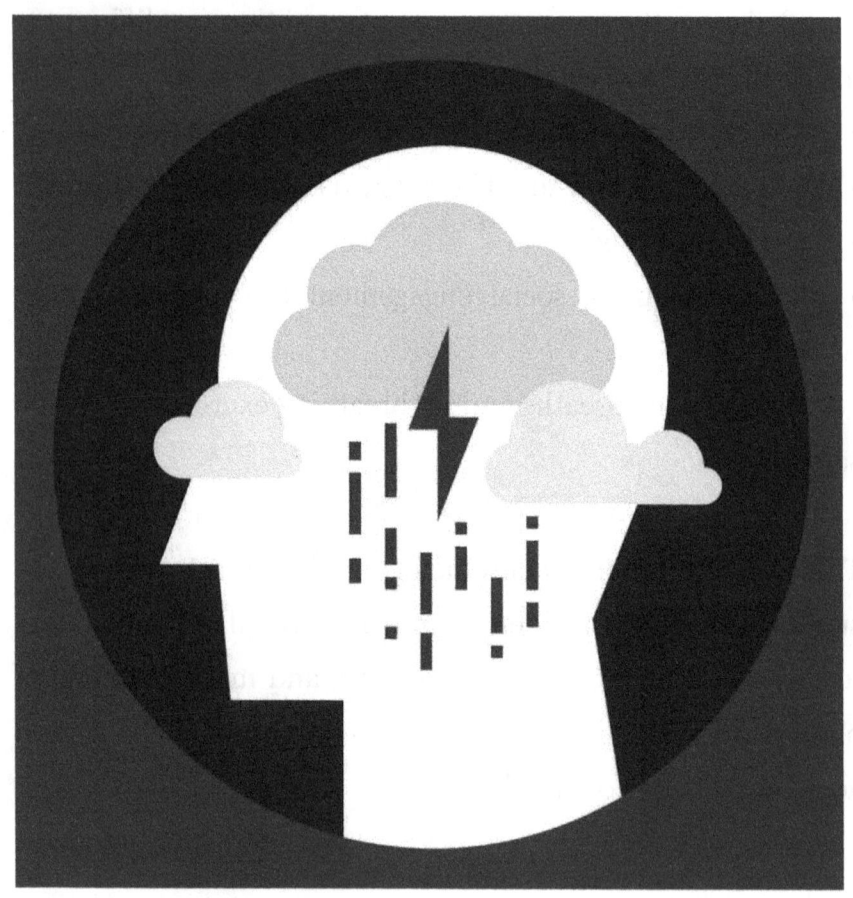

Post-traumatic stress disorder (PTSD) has gained considerable attention in recent years due to its occurrence among military veterans, especially those returning from the long, ongoing conflicts in the Middle East. These traumatized individuals may have experienced severe physical injuries, but in many cases, however, their injuries are psychological, resulting from their overwhelming reactions to their battlefield experiences. In earlier wars, mentally traumatized veterans were suffering from shell shock, the result of seeing and feeling the consequences of war. We now recognize this condition as PTSD.

Typical symptoms of PTSD include flashbacks of the traumatic event or the inability to stop thinking about it obsessively, anxiety, depression, sleeplessness, and recurring nightmares. Beyond the discomforts of experiencing PTSD, it is now known that it can lead to suicidal thoughts and suicidal behavior. In many cases, PTSD can lead to continuing deep depression and anxiety and eating disorders and substance abuse, notably drugs and alcohol.

Apart from veterans, people in all walks of life may have had terrifying, traumatic experiences, either themselves or as witnesses, that trigger PTSD, like an automobile accident, sexual or other physical assault, a serious fall at home, or loss of a loved one. Any of these extremely distressing experiences may initiate the PTSD response. Victims of PTSD may have been told to shape up or get over it, but today, PTSD is a recognized, serious psychological condition requiring professional assistance to resolve. It may affect children as well as adults.

Based on the Polyvagal Theory, many psychologists now believe that PTSD has its roots in the dorsal vagal response of the parasympathetic nervous system. This is the primitive freezing or shutting down mechanism triggered when the person or animal faces an impossible or overwhelming immediate threat. When this dorsal vagal response is initiated, it can cause immobility, speechlessness, fainting, and even severe shock. PTSD appears to be an ongoing form of dorsal vagal reaction.

The Polyvagal Theory's potential treatments for overcoming dorsal vagal-caused PTSD, an understanding of the human brain's evolution and functions are presented for perspective.

The Three-Part Brain

The human brain, with its complexity of 100 billion or so neurons and perhaps 100 trillion neural connections, is generally known to be organized into two hemispheres, the left, recognized for controlling rational, logical, organizational thoughts, and the right, associated with creative, imaginative and unstructured thinking. We also know that the functioning nervous system is comprised of the brain, spinal cord, and between them, the brainstem.

The brain is where all the conscious and unconscious action occurs, from managing our cardiovascular, respiratory, and digestive functions to feelings, senses, and sensations and embracing all thought, memory, and decision-making.

The spinal cord is the central cable that receives all nerve impulses from the extremities and forwards these impulses to the brain and returns the brain's reactions to the impulses with the appropriate reaction.

The brainstem is where 10 of the 12 cranial nerves originate and extend to the organs and other key areas, including number 10, the longest, most diverse neuron, the vagus nerve.

But we know today that the evolution of the human brain has been built upon a sequential three-part structure, beginning with the earliest, most primitive part, called the reptilian brain, then continuing to evolve an early old or paleomammalian brain, and concluding with a more sophisticated new or neo-mammalian brain. Each part has specific functions to perform:

The early reptilian brain is responsible for basic, involuntary reflex actions, including reproduction urges, arousal to a range of stimuli, and maintaining a balanced, normal homeostasis state. It can be considered a fundamental survival mechanism. One of its continuing characteristics is compulsiveness.

The old-mammalian, or paleomammalian brain, is positioned to surround the reptilian brain; it manages emotions, learning, and memory functions. It enabled early mammals to remember and act upon favorable and unfavorable experiences, for example.

The new-mammalian, or neo-mammalian brain, is responsible for conscious thought and self-awareness and is positioned atop the two early brain parts. All of our reasoning, decision-making, and rationalizations occur here.

But one may ask if we evolved from reptiles? The concept of our brains evolving from reptiles comes as a surprise. We understand that we evolved from mammals since we are mammals. Okay, but reptiles? Over the long course of evolution, the earliest mammals evolved from, yes, reptiles, and not from the dinosaurs that became extinct 66 million years ago or the dinosaurs that grew feathers and evolved into birds. Our reptilian ancestors were small and smarter than the large dinosaurs, which gave them an edge in natural selection. They had strong survival skills built into their small but highly functional reptilian brains, and some of these hardy reptiles evolved into small mammals. In their turn, these early mammals evolved more complex brains, the paleomammalian brain, with its added values of learning, memory, and emotion. As mammals further evolved as primates, the third neo-mammalian brain component developed, giving Homo Sapiens the ability to think consciously and with increasing complexity.

The three parts of our current triune brain correspond, approximately, to the brainstem and cerebellum (reptilian), limbic brain, which includes the hippocampus, amygdala, and hypothalamus (paleo mammalian), and the neocortex (neo-mammalian). Because the reptilian-originated brainstem reacts completely unconsciously and immediately for survival, historically, it tends to dominate in many situations when the brain perceives danger or other need for prompt action. The conflict between the purely instinctive reptilian brain and the two more advanced components is considered by some to be represented by Freud's ongoing battles between the conscious and the subconscious.

The complexity of brain functioning begins to become clear. These aspects include the two-hemisphere structure, vertical networks connecting the layers and departments of the brain, and a near-infinite number of interacting neurons and variations in brain structure due to gender, genetic and environmental influences.

In recent times, the precise sequential evolution and functioning of the triune brain and its exclusivity among humans have been questioned by some animal behaviorists since complex brains have developed among non-mammal species, including certain birds. Also, new studies demonstrate that in humans, the prefrontal cortex performs complex functions apart from the neocortex functions.

Post-Traumatic Brain Reeducation

Separate from the psychological disorders associated with PTSD, physical brain injuries are resulting in serious trauma. About 10 million people worldwide suffer traumatic brain injury (TBI) each year, and many cases are fatal, and most who survive the injury experience some degree of cognitive impairment. These traumas may occur in many circumstances, including vehicular accidents, sports injuries, falls inside and outside the home, acts of conflict or violence, even being struck by falling objects.

There is a range of treatments to reverse the impairment, and the type and duration of treatment depend on the type and severity of the trauma. Generally, a multidisciplinary set of treatments is required, involving psychiatric and neurologic medical practices, as well as pharmacotherapy.

Classifying TBI as mild, moderate, or severe depends on several key factors: Degree of post-traumatic consciousness, duration of the coma if experienced by the patient, and the degree and duration of post-traumatic amnesia. Generally, TBI patients whose symptoms continue for one month or more are classified as either moderate or severe and whose full recovery takes years. At the same time, those showing marked improvement within a few weeks are considered mild cases and often return to full cognitive function within two months.

There are several impairments to the cognitive functions following TBI. These are the most commonly treated:

- Decreased ability to concentrate
- Impaired attentiveness
- Reduced visual-spatial cognizance
- The tendency to be easily distracted
- Memory lapses and impairments
- Loss of executive ability (decision-making)
- Disrupted communications skills
- Judgmental lapses and dysfunctions

TBI patients' reeducation begins with assessments based on standardized testing protocols, including visual and auditory attentiveness, visual and verbal measurements, language comprehension and understanding, executive function (decisiveness), overall mental and intellectual function, and motor function.

Post-traumatic brain reeducation is undertaken primarily through cognitive rehabilitation, which increases the injured person's abilities in the processing and interpretation of information and the overall performance of mental functions. Cognitive rehabilitation is most effective in mild or moderate TBI levels and with persons who have a high level of motivation to succeed in the recovery. The multidisciplinary group that collaborates with brain re-educational therapy may include doctors, speech and language specialists, and physical and occupational therapists. However, it is recognized that each patient's treatment will be unique, prescribed, and tailored to each individual, based on the specific injuries suffered and resultant trauma.

One important approach that has wide application is attention process training (ATP), which is based on mental skills training, gradually increasing the exercises' complexity, from simple initially and subsequently increasing in complexity, forcing the brain to retrain itself. The exercises include selective attention, focused attentiveness, alternating attention, divided attentiveness, and sustained attentiveness.

The Parasympathetic Recovery

The Polyvagal Theory links PTSD to one dimension of the parasympathetic nervous system (PNS), the early-evolved dorsal vagal freeze survival mechanism. The dorsal vagal mechanism may protect an animal by allowing it to play dead until the coast is clear. Still, in a human being, it can lead to inaction, inability to think or speak, or worse, passing out or fainting, shock, or even cardiac arrest. With the linking of PTSD to the dorsal vagal mechanism, the unrecognized cause may now be open to evaluation and potentially alleviate the symptoms of PTSD.

Specifically, the other, more recently evolved PNS response, the calming, relaxing, socially engaging ventral vagal response, may be applied to reduce the emotional and physical symptoms of PTSD. The methods used to achieve vagal tone and lower heart rates and breathing rates, reactivate the digestive system, and induce an all-encompassing state of calm and relaxation may be applied by the individual, easily, every day. These methods include meditation, yoga stretches and poses, and managed deep and conscious breathing. The practice of deep, slow breathing, with the forceful extension of the diaphragm to tone the vagus nerve, is applicable as part of meditation or Yoga or simply done without other techniques.

It can also include auricular and facial massage, the vagus nerve's massage as it passes next to the right and left carotid artery in the neck, and cold facial therapy. Mindfulness practice, or being in the moment in which all outside thoughts are prevented from intruding, can also be beneficial. The person concentrates on every external sound, every feeling, and awareness of things in the environment. Vocal stimulation of the vagus nerve can be done easily by singing, gargling, or reciting a mantra while performing mantra and transcendental meditation.

Another application of Polyvagal Theory to treating PTSD is for the individual to recognize that the symptoms of PTSD are biological, caused by the body's primitive instincts and reflexes to protect itself and that the body can be taught to relax, get over it, rejoin, and socially engage with those who are living active, normal lifestyles. This is called somatic awareness, and it trains the individual to become aware of basic bodily functions like heart rate and breathing and consciously try to slow them down. The deep breathing exercises may help achieve a sense of bodily control.

The reduction or elimination of PTSD symptoms can further be achieved by practicing a series of mental exercises called attentional control, a conscious effort to recognize the cues that may trigger PTSD reactions, and gently but firmly cancel them out by acknowledging that there is no danger, nothing to fear, and all are well. This form of body awareness is called cognitive behavior therapy (CBT). It encourages the individual to be aware that an unneeded fight or flight response is continuing and can be shut down by conscious thought, replacing disturbing thoughts and memories with relaxing, peaceful thoughts. Over time and with practice, replacing bad thoughts with positive ones will make the cooling down of the dorsal vagal action-orientation easier.

Reading Body Language

Body language has long been associated with a few popular positions and movements that are believed to be subconscious cues as to a person's true meaning or intentions—for example, having one's arms crossed signals a negative interest in what is being said, or a hand over one's mouth while speaking may be a sign of a lie being told. Unconsciously nodding one's head indicates agreement; a handshake suggests the type of character, depending on whether it is firm or weak, and if eye contact is maintained or not. In reality, most of these body language cues are anecdotal and may have some basis, or they may not.

But Polyvagal Theory has shed new light on body language, on multiple levels, by revealing one's interest in a social engagement, for example, or sending a signal that can trigger social engagement or other interaction in the second person, who may, in turn, respond with their body language subconsciously. The use of facial expressions to elicit various types of responses is being used to communicate and engage with autistic children, in testimony to this approach's effectiveness. (Communicating and engaging with autistic children)

Do the popular body language signals mean anything, or are they, as implied above, merely anecdotal, believed, and circulated but without substantiation? A study conducted by UCLA found that only 7% of what is said is believed or acknowledged, based only on the words spoken. The tonality of the speaker's voice accounts for 38% of communications, leaving 50% of communications based on body language, gestures, and expressions.

Resistance to what is being said or shown is frequently shown by crossed arms and crossed legs.

A smile is not sincere when it is limited to the mouth, whereas a sincere smile engages more of the face, including crinkling the eyes.

Mirroring or imitating your body positions signifies that the other person agrees with what you are saying or proposing.

Power positions radiate a sense of command or control. A person who assumes control will tend to stand upright, extend arms, and otherwise occupy more space in a room. This type of person is encouraging interaction or possibly engagement.

Eye contact is not always synonymous with engagement or interest because extended or prolonged eye contact may be forced or deliberate, suggesting the person is hiding a true intention.

Discomfort or surprise may cause raised eyebrows. Conversely, a truly interested person will not tend to raise their eyebrows when spoken to, except to acknowledge an exceptionally unusual remark.

Nodding is positive, except when it's exaggerated because too much nodding suggests discomfort with what is being said.

Tension signals stress. A furrowed brow tightened neck muscles, or a clenched jaw may signify that what is being said makes the person uncomfortable.

Are these findings valid? It's probably to some degree, but it's important to realize that the subject of body language has been debated for decades. As a result, many people you may be speaking with, or meet in an interview, maybe consciously nodding or smiling or firmly shaking your hand, deliberately trying to make a good impression. You, in turn, might consider your body language and try not to send the wrong message.

Effect of Trauma On Nervous System And Its Response

If we have an uncertain injury from quite a while ago, we may live in the form of never-ending battle or-flight. We might have the option to channel this battle or-flight tension into exercises, for example, cleaning the house, raking the forgets about, or working at the rec center. Yet, these exercises will have an unexpected vibe compared to what they would if they were finished with social commitment science (think "Whistle While You Work").

For some injury survivors, no movement effectively channels their battle or-flight sensations. Subsequently, they feel caught, and their bodies shut down. These customers may live in a variant of the ceaseless shutdown.

Diminish Levine, a long-lasting companion, and associate of Porges, has examined the shutdown reaction through creature perceptions and bodywork with customers. In Waking the Tiger: Healing Trauma, he clarifies that rising out of shutdown requires a shiver or shake to release suspended battle or-flight vitality. In a dangerous circumstance, on the off chance that we have shut down and an open door for dynamic endurance introduces itself, we can wake ourselves up. As advocates, we may perceive this move from shutdown to battle or-trip in a customer's move from the gloom into nervousness.

In any case, how might we help our customers move into their social commitment science? On the off chance that customers live in a progressively dissociative, discouraged, shutdown way, we should assist them with moving incidentally into battle or-flight. As customers experience a battle or-flight force, we should then assist them with finding a feeling of wellbeing. When they can detect that they are protected, they can move into their social commitment framework.

The body-mindfulness systems that are a piece of intellectual conduct treatment (CBT) and argumentative conduct treatment (DBT) can assist customers with moving out of dissociative, shutdown reactions by urging them to turn out to be increasingly epitomized. When customers are increasingly present in their bodies and better ready to take care of flashing strong strain, they can wake up from a shutdown reaction. As customers actuate out of shutdown and move toward battle or-flight sensations, the idea rebuilding methods that are likewise part of CBT and DBT can instruct customers to assess their wellbeing all the more precisely. Intelligent listening methods can assist customers with feeling an association with their advisors. This causes it workable for these customers to feel sufficiently safe to move into social commitment science.

The polyvagal hypothesis gives a hypothetical stage to decipher social conduct inside a neurophysiological setting. The accentuation on phylogeny gives an arranging rule to comprehend the progressive succession of versatile reactions. The social commitment framework not just furnishes direct social contact with others but also tweaks physiological state to positively influence social conduct by applying an inhibitory impact on the thoughtful sensory system. From the polyvagal hypothesis point of view, social conduct is a new property of the autonomic sensory system's phylogenetic advancement. Reliable with this progressive model saw difficulties to endurance regularly bring about a neural disintegration from the later frameworks of positive social conduct and social correspondence to the more crude fight! Flight and shirking frameworks. The hypothesis leads not exclusively to the clarification of the pathophysiological states related to different clinical disarranges yet additionally bolsters the presentation of another worldview that may have general applications for people with troubles in social conduct

Conclusion

Thank you for reading through the end of Polyvagal theory book. Hopefully, it was a book full of information that was useful and relevant to you while delivered in a method that was readily understood. Our bodies, when faced with fear and anxiety, it responds to the situation through the vagus nerve activation. There is the modern fight or flight response, in which the body sees some sort of stressor and is convinced that it can fend it off in some way, shape, or form, either in fighting or running away. This is why you get afraid or angry when you are stressed out. Finally, the state of mind in which you are calm and ready to socialize is known as the connection state of mind. This is where you can make meaningful interactions and connections with other people.

The polyvagal approach recommends that it is essential, not exclusively, to comprehend the vagal efferent activities on the heart from a neurophysiological degree of request. Yet, the versatile capacity of neural regulation of the heart must be interpreted inside the setting of the phylogeny of the autonomic nervous system. In the areas over, a few control discipline myths have been deconstructed and interpreted depending on the inquiry level. These centers outline detailed explanations to stimulate further logical experiments and challenges using well-designed structured investigations.

In any case, when research techniques depend on a neurophysiological degree of inquiry, at that point, the mission for a component of cardiac vagal tone is refined to concentrate on strategies that individually measure every one of the two vagal systems. The last methodology should be expressed to psych physiologists since the two vagal systems advanced to help various types of behavior.

Vagal activity starting in the nucleus ambiguous is neurophysiological and neuroanatomical connected to regulating the striated muscles of the face and head, structures that are engaged with social communication and emotions. Hypothetically, RSA should intently resemble individual and intra-singular varieties in emotion connection, social interaction, and behavioral status.

Interestingly, vagal action beginning in the DMX ought to reflect tonic impacts to the visceral organs (i.e., basically subdiaphragmatic). The quick and immense increase in the DMX output that may deliver bradycardia, apnea, or defecation would happen as a defense procedure to decrease metabolic demands. Maybe, the negative feature of stress and well-being defenselessness being related to the slower rhythms may have driven researchers to accept that these rhythms were affected by the sympathetic sensory system.

The polyvagal perspective shifts the research from theoretical techniques towards hypothesis-driven ideal models subordinates upon specific neural mechanisms. Preeminent, the polyvagal theory accentuates the significance of phylogenetic changes in the neural structures controlling the autonomic nervous system. The phylogenetic technique gives experiences into the versatile capacity and the neural regulation of the two vagal systems. Without having constructs from the Polyvagal Theory to depict versatile abilities and decide the two vagal systems' estimation details.

One related with calm states and social commitment manners and the other a minimal defense system that is conceivably bad to warm-blooded animals. It would not be conceivable to explain the methods and components of the cardiovascular vagal tone segments.

www.ingramcontent.com/pod-product-compliance
Lightning Source LLC
Chambersburg PA
CBHW071115030426
42336CB00013BA/2093